Understanding Why Addicts Are Not All Alike

Understanding Why Addicts Are Not All Alike

Recognizing the Types and How Their Differences Affect Intervention and Treatment

Gary L. Fisher

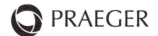 PRAEGER

AN IMPRINT OF ABC-CLIO, LLC
Santa Barbara, California • Denver, Colorado • Oxford, England

Library of Congress Cataloging-in-Publication Data

Fisher, Gary L.
    Understanding why addicts are not all alike : recognizing the types and how their differences affect intervention and treatment / Gary L. Fisher.
        p. ; cm.
    Includes bibliographical references and index.
    ISBN 978–0–313–38707–4 (hard copy : alk. paper) — ISBN 978–0–313–38708–1 (ebook)
1. Substance abuse—Patients—Classification. 2. Substance abuse—Patients—Rehabilitation.
I. Title.
    [DNLM: 1. Substance-Related Disorders—psychology. 2. Substance-Related Disorders—therapy. 3. Behavior, Addictive—classification. 4. Behavior, Addictive—psychology. 5. Models, Psychological. 6. Treatment Outcome. WM 270]
RC564.F574   2011
362.29—dc22   2011009439

ISBN: 978–0–313–38707–4
EISBN: 978–0–313–38708–1

15 14 13 12 11   1 2 3 4 5

This book is also available on the World Wide Web as an eBook.
Visit www.abc-clio.com for details.

Praeger
An Imprint of ABC-CLIO, LLC

ABC-CLIO, LLC
130 Cremona Drive, P.O. Box 1911
Santa Barbara, California 93116-1911

This book is printed on acid-free paper ∞

Manufactured in the United States of America

To all addicts, those in recovery and those still searching

Contents

Preface

As an academic discipline, the field of alcohol and other drug addiction treatment is relatively young. The first treatment program that had some resemblance to the treatment programs we see today was developed by the Hazeldon Foundation in the 1940s and 1950s. There was not much of a research base for the development of this program and it was designed for alcoholics only. During the Vietnam War, there was a concern among the military and government administration officials about the number of returning soldiers addicted to heroin. A physician from Chicago, Dr. Jerry Jaffee, became involved in treating these veterans, primarily through methadone maintenance. Dr. Jaffee attracted residents who were interested in treating drug addicts and a specialty in addiction medicine occurred. As with most medical specialties, this also spurred academic research, in this case, in addiction. Dr. Jaffee became the nation's first drug czar during the Nixon Administration. In 1993, he was an administrator in the federal Center for Substance Abuse Treatment (part of the Health and Human Services' Substance Abuse and Mental Health Services Administration). By then, Jaffee had realized that the addiction treatment field would never apply the research findings coming out of colleges and universities unless the education and training for treatment providers was upgraded. Up to that time, nearly all drug and alcohol counselors were recovering individuals, and states required very little, if any, education and training. Because of a federal grant initiative (still going on today) that Jaffee started, training programs for addiction-treatment providers were started in colleges and universities across the country, at both the undergraduate and graduate levels. States were encouraged to increase their requirements for certification or licensure to become a drug and alcohol counselor. Public-sector treatment programs (treatment programs financed with federal dollars) were incentivized to incorporate evidence-based practices in their programs. In addition, pre-service and in-service professionals in related disciplines (e.g., social work, nursing, mental health counseling, medicine) were provided training in the latest research on assessment and treatment. All of these efforts have been successful in improving the education and training of addiction-treatment providers and related professionals and in enhancing the practices in treatment programs.

However, this level of attention to improving addiction treatment has only been underway for 17 years. That is really not a very long time compared to the long histories of mental health and medical treatment. Furthermore, there is institutional resistance to change. In the mid-1990s, I was in charge of an organization that was contracted by the state to put on an annual summer institute for the prevention and treatment community in our state. The state agency wanted to use the event to encourage treatment programs to use evidence-based strategies. We had a session on methadone maintenance treatment for heroin addicts. This type of treatment has one of the best outcomes of any type of addiction treatment. A long-time treatment director for a large public sector program in the state who was a recovering addict stormed out in the middle of the session and told me, "I'm not going to listen to any of that f—ing s—t." He firmly believed in a strict abstinence model of treatment, and he was not open to any information that was not consistent with this point of view. Because of the long history in addiction treatment of utilizing recovering individuals who had no formal training as treatment providers, there was a tendency for treatment programs to adopt a very rigid concept of treatment. It was analogous to a religious group that preaches that there is only one way to salvation—their way. In no way am I denigrating treatment providers who are recovering. I have been training addiction-treatment counselors for many years and the best ones I have ever worked with are recovering individuals who get formal training. But, recovering counselors without training only have their personal experience to use and the tendency is to apply that experience to every patient.

So, although the addiction field has come a long way, there are still many ways of looking at addiction and many ways of treating addiction that are based on old models and have not been revised to reflect research and the reality of the population in treatment today. When the Hazeldon Foundation started its treatment program, the patient population consisted of mainly white, middle-class, alcoholic men. It is a little hard to justify using the same methods today when the patient population contains males and females; adolescents through senior citizens; every socio-economic, ethnic, and racial group you can name; patients with co-occurring mental disorders; people with HIV and hepatitis; the homeless; criminal justice populations; persons with disabilities; and patients who use alcohol and many other drugs. That is not to imply that there aren't many treatment programs across the country that have implemented the most up-to-date evidence-based practices and that have a well-trained workforce. But, as will be seen in the first chapter of this book, there still is a lot of data that shows that treatment could be improved.

This book is an attempt in that direction. It is an effort to explain some of the results seen in treatment-outcome studies and to challenge some of the assumptions that many in the addiction field routinely make. When you read about the data on treatment, you will see that it is imperative that we intervene earlier with those who are beginning to have problems with alcohol and other drugs, get more people into treatment who have serious substance use problems, keep people in treatment longer, and manage treatment and post-treatment recovery more effectively. I hope this information helps move the field in that direction.

Case examples are used in Chapters 2, 3, and 4 to illustrate the concepts discussed. But, case examples are not proof of anything. They may or may not be typical. The cases were not scientifically chosen. Through a variety of means, I was able to find individuals who seemed to effectively illustrate the concepts I was presenting and who were willing to either be interviewed or to write their story. In order to protect everyone's anonymity, I do not say how I came in contact with the individuals, how I came to know them, or how I obtained information that is not included in their interview or story. Every name is changed to minimize the possibility of identification.

My caution with case examples arises from the way that such cases are used by people to "prove" a point. For example, one of the cases in the disease model chapter achieved long-term sobriety by attending Alcoholics Anonymous and never participated in formal treatment. That doesn't prove that treatment is unnecessary or that AA works for everyone. If you work long enough in the addiction-treatment field you will find examples of nearly everything. I know someone who was a heroin addict and served time in federal prison. His treatment was a religious-based program that does not use any of the principles commonly used in public sector treatment programs. He has been clean from illicit drug use for decades and is a model citizen. But, he drinks alcohol moderately. That is considered impossible by people who adhere to the disease model of addiction. A man I knew (now deceased) was a disease model alcoholic who was nearly dead when he went to treatment. He attended a residential program many years ago that gave patients a drug that made them very nauseous when combined with alcohol and then they made the patients drink. He stayed sober until his death and never attended an AA meeting. You would be hard pressed to find a treatment provider or researcher who would predict that such a program would produce long-term sobriety. A former president (George W. Bush) describes his drinking (which was alcoholic) and how he got sober through attendance at church and through his faith. There are many ways addicts get sober. The point is that the cases make the concepts discussed concrete, they are interesting, and they contain elements that lead to other issues I want to illustrate. However, the only thing they are evidence of is that there are addicts who fit the subtypes being discussed.

It is typical at this point to thank people who have helped create this work. I do want to acknowledge those individuals who shared their stories through interviews or their writing. However, I can't tell you their real names. As for others, I really kept this project to myself. When I was asked what I was working on, I would usually say, "It's just an academic book about addicts. It's too boring to talk about." This need for secrecy may be my own paranoia but I wanted to fiercely guard that anonymity of the people in the case examples. I do want to thank my editor, Debbie Carvalko. This is the second book Debbie has worked on with me and she had to show a great deal of patience on this one. I was running for an elective office through nearly all of 2010 and I moved the deadline a couple of times. Fortunately for this book, I lost the election and could devote the time needed to complete it. Finally, I want to mention my wonderful wife Carole (who knows very little about this project); my adult children Colin, Jacob, Brooke, and Aaron (who know less than Carole); and my grandchildren Kaya and Miles (who are too young to care). But, they all like to see their names in my books.

For those readers who do not have a great deal of background or experience in this field, there are appendices on classification of drugs and treatment approaches and strategies. The appendix on classification of drugs groups mind-altering substances (including alcohol) by their effect on the central nervous system. For each classification, there is information on the formal and slang terms for the various substances in that group; signs of intoxication, overdose, tolerance, and withdrawal; and acute and chronic effects of the drugs. The appendix on treatment approaches and strategies describes what actually happens in addiction treatment programs. If you are not familiar with the addiction field, reading these two appendices before you read the rest of the book should provide you with enough information to fully grasp the material in each chapter. The final appendix contains Internet and hard copy resources on the addiction field in general and on specific topics related to concepts discussed in the book. This appendix is not intended to be an exhaustive list but it will provide a starting place for thorough research on nearly any topic in the addiction field.

ONE

Addicts: Who They Are, What They Do

Each year, the federal government conducts a survey, the National Survey on Drug Use & Health, to gather information on the prevalence, patterns, and consequences of tobacco, alcohol, and other drug use of Americans ages 12 and older. In 2009 (the most recent data available), the results indicated that there were an estimated 22.5 million Americans who could be classified as having a substance abuse or substance dependence disorder.[1] This number has remained very stable since 2002, the first year that accurate comparisons year to year can be made. These 22.5 million people would fit the diagnostic criteria that behavioral healthcare professionals (i.e., psychiatrists, psychologists, social workers, mental health counselors, and drug and alcohol counselors) use to decide who needs treatment for an alcohol and/or other drug problem. However, in 2009, only 2.6 million people received treatment for an alcohol and/or other drug problem, according to this same survey.[2] Therefore, based on this survey, there would seem to be nearly 20 million people who need treatment but do not receive it. Most research articles and books focus on those people who get treatment for an alcohol and/or other drug problem. This book discusses all of the individuals with substance use disorders; those who receive treatment and those who do not. Why is that important? There are 10 times the number of people who have problems with alcohol and/or other drugs who don't receive any help compared to those who do receive help. As will be shown in this chapter, substance use disorders cause individuals, families, and society numerous problems and cost all of us a tremendous amount of money. So, it makes sense to understand why most people with these problems fail to get treatment and whether there is anything that can be done (or should be done) to change this situation.

NOMENCLATURE

Before proceeding, it is important to understand the terms that will be used in this book to describe the conditions that will be discussed. Terminology can be challenging in this field. When the phrase "alcohol and other drugs" is used, the intent is to be sure that readers understand that alcohol is a drug and it is a drug that people can have problems with. "Other drugs" include substances that are currently illegal in all or most circumstances (e.g., heroin, cocaine, methamphetamine, marijuana) and legal substances that can be used illicitly (e.g., prescription drugs).

"Substance use disorders" refer to conditions in the *Diagnostic and Statistical Manual of Mental Disorders, Fourth Edition, Text Revision* (DSM-IV TR), the "bible" used by behavioral healthcare professionals to diagnose a wide variety of mental health problems. There are two substance use disorders: Substance Abuse Disorders and Substance Dependence Disorders, and there are specific criteria to diagnose these conditions. The Criteria for Substance Abuse in the DSM-IV TR are as follows:

A. A maladaptive pattern of substance use leading to clinically significant impairment or distress, as manifested by one (or more) of the following, occurring within a 12-month period:
   (1) recurrent substance use resulting in a failure to fulfill major role obligations at work, school, or home (e.g., repeated absences or poor work performance related to substance use, substance-related absences or poor work performance related to substance use, substance-related absences, suspensions, or expulsions from school, neglect of children or household)
   (2) recurrent substance use in situations in which it is physically hazardous (e.g., driving an automobile or operating a machine when impaired by substance use)
   (3) recurrent substance-related legal problems (e.g., arrests for substance-related disorderly conduct)
   (4) continued substance use despite having persistent or recurrent social or interpersonal problems caused or exacerbated by the effects of the substance (e.g., arguments with spouse about consequences of intoxication, physical fights)

B. The symptoms have never met the criteria for Substance Dependence for this class of substance.[3]*

In simple terms, the criteria for diagnosis of a substance abuse disorder means that a person has encountered "trouble" as a result of alcohol or other drug use. "Trouble" may involve work, school, or home responsibilities; contact with the criminal justice system; or relationships with friends, family members, co-workers, or strangers. The terms "persistent" and/or "recurrent" are used in each of the criteria to differentiate the person who had too much to drink at the company Christmas party and got into an argument with his girlfriend from people who demonstrate consistent problems. In other words, people who experience a one-time occurrence of "trouble" would not be diagnosed with a substance abuse disorder.

It is important to remember that whatever kind of "trouble" that occurs, the persistent or recurrent events must occur within a 12-month period. So, if you always miss work the Monday following the Super Bowl because of a hangover, you would not meet the criteria for a substance abuse disorder, that is unless you are also calling in periodically after Monday-night football. As specified in "B," a person cannot be diagnosed with a substance abuse disorder for a drug (e.g., cocaine) if that person can be diagnosed with a substance dependence disorder for the same class of drugs (i.e., other central nervous system stimulants such as methamphetamine).

The Criteria for Substance Dependence in the DSM-IV TR are as follows:

A maladaptive pattern of substance use, leading to clinically significant impairment or distress, as manifested by three (or more) of the following, occurring at any time in the same 12-month period:

(1) tolerance, as defined by either of the following:
  (a) a need for markedly increased amounts of the substance to achieve intoxication or desired effect
  (b) markedly diminished effect with continued use of the same amount of the substance
(2) withdrawal, as manifested by either of the following:
  (a) the characteristic withdrawal syndrome for the substance . . .
  (b) the same (or a closely related) substance is taken to relieve or avoid withdrawal symptoms

---

*Reprinted with permission from the *Diagnostic and Statistical Manual of Mental Disorders, Text Revision, Fourth Edition* (Copyright 2000). American Psychiatric Association.

(3) the substance is often taken in larger amounts or over a longer period than was intended

(4) there is a persistent desire or unsuccessful efforts to cut down or control substance use

(5) a great deal of time is spent in activities necessary to obtain the substance (e.g., visiting multiple doctors or driving long distances), use the substance (e.g., chain-smoking), or recover from its effects

(6) important social, occupational, or recreational activities are given up or reduced because of substance use

(7) the substance use is continued despite knowledge of having a persistent or recurrent physical or psychological problem that is likely to have been caused or exacerbated by the substance (e.g., current cocaine use despite recognition of cocaine-induced depression, or continued drinking despite recognition that an ulcer was made worse by alcohol consumption)[4][†]

If substance abuse could be simplified as "trouble," substance dependence can be called "serious trouble." When trying to help prospective counselors understand these diagnostic categories, we often describe substance abuse as continuing to use alcohol or other drugs in spite of consequences and substance dependence as continuing to use alcohol or other drugs regardless of the consequences. Obviously, a substance dependence disorder is considered to be a more serious condition than a substance abuse disorder, which can be inferred from the nature of the criteria for a substance dependence disorder and the fact that three of the criteria must occur in a 12-month period (as opposed to one criterion for a substance abuse disorder). The first two criteria for a substance dependence disorder (tolerance and withdrawal) historically have been used to differentiate a substance abuse disorder from a substance dependence disorder. In fact, in earlier versions of the *Diagnostic and Statistical Manual of Mental Disorders*, tolerance and withdrawal had to be demonstrated before a diagnosis of a substance dependence disorder could be made. As it was determined that certain classifications of drugs (e.g., hallucinogens) did not result in tolerance or withdrawal but could cause significant life problems, the most recent versions of the manual do not require that tolerance and withdrawal be present. However, both of these characteristics are often seen in people with a substance dependence disorder.

[†]Reprinted with permission from the *Diagnostic and Statistical Manual of Mental Disorders, Text Revision, Fourth Edition* (Copyright 2000). American Psychiatric Association.

Many people know someone who has developed a tolerance to alcohol. We generally say that such a person can "sure hold his booze," and this person may even be admired by peers. Tolerance has been demonstrated with most other classifications of drugs, including marijuana. The body becomes accustomed to alcohol or other drugs and adapts so more and more of the substance must be taken to achieve the desired level of intoxication. As tolerance progresses, the person may need alcohol or other drugs simply to feel normal.

Nearly everyone is familiar with the withdrawal syndrome that occurs in heroin addicts. These symptoms have been graphically depicted in movies and certainly are extremely unpleasant (similar to a bad case of the flu). However, a withdrawal syndrome can be observed with most classifications of drugs and can range from medically dangerous (e.g., alcohol and other central nervous system depressants), to unpleasant and long-lasting (e.g., cocaine and methamphetamine), to mild and short (e.g., marijuana). During medical detoxification from alcohol, patients are usually given some type of minor tranquilizer (e.g., Valium, Ativan) to minimize the severity of the withdrawal from alcohol. Both alcohol and minor tranquilizers are central nervous system depressants. Similarly, heroin addicts can relieve the symptoms of withdrawal by taking prescription pain medication (e.g., Loratab, Vicodin) because these drugs are all opioids.

When a diagnosis of a substance use disorder is made, the substances that are a problem are specified. For example, a person might be diagnosed with an Alcohol Dependence Disorder or a Cannabis (marijuana) Abuse Disorder. There is also "Polysubstance Dependence" that is used when someone can be diagnosed with substance dependence disorders for two different classifications of drugs (e.g., opioids such as heroin and a stimulant such as cocaine).

"Addict" and "addiction" are not terms that are used by professionals to diagnose substance use disorders but are widely used by the general public. Most people probably think of "addict" in relation to people who have a substance dependence disorder on drugs like heroin, cocaine, and methamphetamine, but addict can refer to a substance use disorder for any drug, including alcohol. "Alcoholic" means a person with a substance use disorder involving alcohol. Since most people today use a variety of different drugs, the term "addict" or "addiction" will generally be used to refer to all substance use disorders, including alcohol use disorders.

If you don't have a lot of experience with this field, you may struggle a bit with the term "addict" as it is applied to individuals with substance abuse disorders and who don't use the type of drugs many people associate with addiction (e.g., heroin, cocaine, methamphetamine). For example, later in the book, the case of a person who only uses marijuana is described. Remember that the term "addict" will be used to refer to anyone who can be diagnosed with either a substance abuse or a substance dependence disorder. In other words, there is no judgment or stereotype implied in the use of the term "addict"; it is simply used as a way to generically describe those who have a substance use disorder.

THE IMPORTANCE OF EXAMINING ALL ADDICTS, INCLUDING THOSE NOT RECEIVING TREATMENT

Addicts cause of a lot of problems. They utilize healthcare resources (especially emergency room services) as a result of accidents, injuries, and illnesses; have high rates of unemployment and underemployment; impact the criminal justice system; and disrupt their families. The costs of these problems have been estimated to be over $500 billion per year, with more than 123,000 annual deaths as a result of alcohol and other drug abuse.[5] According to a study conducted by the National Center on Addiction and Substance Abuse at Columbia University, the federal government spends 9.6% of its budget and state governments spend 15.7% of their budgets on substance abuse and addiction. Fifty-eight percent of this spending is on health care and 13.1% is spent on criminal justice (i.e., incarceration, parole, probation, and criminal, juvenile, and family courts). Appallingly, for every dollar federal, state, and local governments spend on prevention and treatment, they spend nearly $60 on the consequences of substance abuse and addiction.[6]

With these enormous costs, it makes sense to do something with addicts to ameliorate these problems. There is evidence that substance abuse treatment has positive effects on healthcare costs, employment, law-enforcement involvement, and other areas.[7] However, there are also many problems with the treatment system. In 2006 (most recent data available), only 47.5% of those who entered treatment completed it.[8] Over half of those who went to treatment had one or more previous treatment episodes.[9] To be fair, this is not different than what happens in treating many chronic health conditions, such as hypertension, diabetes, and asthma (i.e., some patients not complying with treatment recommendations and relapses). But, the fact remains that most people with substance use disorders who receive treatment do not complete it, and most require more than one treatment episode. There are many other problems with treatment, including the training and credentials of treatment providers, lack of services for people with co-occurring mental health disorders, lack of services designed for specific populations (e.g., adolescents, women, minorities, elderly), inadequate duration of treatment, and minimal post-treatment follow-up. However, for the purposes of this book, we will focus on the causes for low treatment completion and multiple treatment episodes. Much more will be said about these topics.

So we know that, of the 2.6 million addicts who receive treatment each year, about half complete treatment. Therefore, about 1.3 million addicts out of the 22.5 million who need treatment actually finish their program. That is less than 6%. Regardless of how good or bad treatment is or how many problems exist in the treatment system, the major problem is that the vast majority of addicts do not get to treatment. Why is that?

First of all, results from the National Household Survey showed that the vast majority (95%) of those people who needed treatment but didn't get it did not feel they needed it.[10] That finding is not surprising to behavioral healthcare professionals, who frequently encounter resistance to treatment from clients who are seen as having a substance use disorder. For those who felt they needed treatment but did not receive it, the primary reasons given were lack of health coverage and could not afford the cost (36.8%), not ready to stop using (30.5%), could handle the problem without treatment (10.2%), no transportation/inconvenient (9.7%), had health coverage but did not cover treatment or did not cover cost (8.8%), might have negative effect on job (8.6%), and might cause neighbors/community to have negative opinion (8.5%).[11‡] So, even among the small proportion of those who admit to having a problem, nearly one-third are simply not ready to discontinue their alcohol and other drug use.

These findings have not escaped the attention of federal officials who are responsible for substance abuse treatment policies. There have been a lot of resources devoted to early screening and intervention and the utilization of evidence-based strategies to motivate addicts to enter treatment. However, there has not been much progress in moving more addicts into treatment.

If you are not a behavioral healthcare professional, you might be wondering why so many addicts are not interested in treatment. The analogy I use to explain this phenomenon is to consider a situation where you are in love with someone but your family and friends do not approve. When your family and friends try to talk to you about your lover, you are completely resistant to their efforts. In your mind, no one can understand your relationship, they must all be jealous, and you can't imagine living

‡Percentages add up to more than 100 because respondents were allowed to name more than one reason.

without this person. You may even continue to cling to the relationship after there is evidence, such as abuse or infidelity, that your lover isn't as wonderful as you thought. Of course, after the relationship ends, you understand what everyone was saying to you. Well, addicts are in a primary, intimate relationship, much like that of a lover, with alcohol and other drugs. It is very difficult to directly confront this relationship in spite of the problems the relationship may be causing. You have probably heard that addicts have to "hit bottom" before they are ready to get help. Although there really isn't evidence to support this generalization, it does make sense to think that many addicts have to encounter some very significant problems before they are willing to commit to treatment.

The discussion thus far demonstrates that it is futile (and probably misleading) to understand addicts by only studying those who enter treatment. That population of addicts is amazingly small compared to the total number of addicts. However, most of what professionals know about addicts is based on this small minority who enter treatment. In addition, the treatment system has functioned as if the treatment population of addicts was all alike and could all be treated the same. In the early days of treatment, most patients were white, male, middle-aged alcoholics. Treatment generally was conducted in residential settings, lasted 28 days, and utilized an orientation based on Alcoholic Anonymous' Twelve Steps. Treatment providers were recovering alcoholics who had little if any formal counselor training. Today, the treatment population is just as diverse as our country's population. Clients usually have problems with multiple drugs (including alcohol); include men and women, adolescents, adults, seniors, every ethnic and racial group; have co-occurring mental disorders (e.g., depression, post-traumatic stress disorder); and may have physical or mental disabilities. Treatment usually occurs in outpatient settings. Logically, every client should have an individualized treatment plan to meet that client's unique needs. However, the treatment system has been slow to adapt to a changing treatment population, and most programs continue to utilize the same old methods for everyone. While there have been and continue to be efforts at the federal and state levels to integrate evidence-based strategies in treatment, these systems are resistant to change.

Ironically, for about a half of century there has been ample evidence that addicts are not all alike, even when the treatment population was much more homogenous in terms of demographic characteristics than it is now. Apart from the obvious observation that people are unique, authors and researchers in the field have described subtypes of addicts; groups that share certain characteristics that are relevant to their treatment. The premise of this book is that these subtypes help explain why so many addicts are not in treatment and why so many addicts in treatment do not complete treatment and require multiple treatment episodes. That is not to say that treatment providers can ignore individual characteristics and needs in developing treatment plans. Clearly, when you are working with an addict at the individual level, these components are important. However, because only about 6% of addicts actually enter and complete treatment, there is a need to examine factors that may explain the behavior of large subgroups of addicts who do not seek treatment or who do not complete it. Given the enormous social costs of addiction, a conceptualization that leads to more effective interventions with addicts is essential.

HISTORY OF SUBTYPES

In 1960, E. M. Jellinek published *The Disease Concept of Alcoholism*,[12] a book that is credited with beginning a conceptualization of addiction that has had profound effects on the field of addiction treatment (the Disease Model of Addiction is thoroughly discussed in the next chapter). However, what is generally not attended to in this seminal work is that Jellinek described five types of alcoholism, only two of which he thought were consistent with his concept of disease. Jellinek used the Greek alphabet to refer to the five types of alcoholics, with Gamma alcoholics (garden-variety alcoholics) and Delta alcoholics (maintenance drinkers) representing the disease types. Alpha alcoholics were described as psychologically dependent on alcohol, Beta alcoholics as having physical consequences from long-term, heavy alcohol use but no psychological or physical dependence, and Epsilon alcoholics as binge drinkers.

Following Jellinek's work, there have been many efforts by scholars to subtype addicts, particularly alcoholics. For those who are interested in the details of the subtyping literature, an article by Lorenzo Leggio and his colleagues provides an excellent review.[13] Two of the earliest typologies were developed by Robert Cloninger and colleagues in 1981 and by Thomas Babor and colleagues in 1992. Both of these schemes were binary classifications. Cloninger's Type 1 was characterized by later onset in life (after age 25), as affecting men and women equally, and as responding relatively well to treatment. Type II alcoholism was characterized by an early onset in life, a presumed inheritance of the condition, as affecting primarily men, and as having a poor response to treatment. Babor's classifications (called Type A and Type B) were similar to Cloninger's but were developed through statistical analysis, while Cloninger's were conceptualized.

With the widespread use of sophisticated statistical techniques, more complex subtyping schemes were developed by a number of researchers. Three, four, and five subtypes were identified in the literature. While Cloninger's early- and late-onset types continued to be identified by many of these scholars, typologies also identified polydrug use, co-occurring mental disorders, and antisocial behavior as characteristics of different subtypes. There have also been efforts to apply subtyping schemes to addicts other than alcoholics. What is consistent among the many different types of subtyping is that treatment populations were always used to establish the subtypes.

However, a study published by researchers associated with the federal government's National Institute on Alcohol Abuse and Alcoholism used statistical methods to subtype nearly 1,500 alcoholics identified through the 2001–2002 National Epidemiological Survey on Alcohol and Related Conditions (NESARC).[14] This was the first and only subtyping research that did not limit the study population to those in treatment. As described by the researchers, "the NESARC sample represents the civilian, non-institutionalized adult population of the United States, including all 50 states and the District of Columbia. It includes persons living in households, military personnel living off-base, and persons residing in boarding or rooming houses, non-transient hotels and motels, shelters, college quarters and group homes."[15] Out of more than 43,000 people surveyed, nearly 1,500 met the criteria for an alcohol use disorder (alcohol abuse or alcohol dependence) in the previous year. Over two-thirds of the sample were male and 71% were Caucasian. The researchers gathered information on the age of onset (age at which the alcohol use disorder first was present), family history of alcohol use disorders, the presence of any co-occurring mental disorders (e.g., depression, post-traumatic stress disorder, personality disorders), the presence of other substance use disorders and behaviors, and involvement in antisocial behaviors. Using sophisticated statistical analyses, the researchers identified five subtypes of alcohol use disorders. Since these subtypes are crucial in understanding the following chapters in this book, each one will be described in detail.

YOUNG ADULT SUBTYPE

As the title of the subtype implies, this group was characterized by their relative youth, with an average age of 24½ years. Their age of onset was also early, a little more than 19½ years of age. What is surprising about the young adult subtype is that it was the largest subtype, composing 31.5% of the total sample of people with alcohol use disorders. Most people tend to think of alcoholics as older than this group. The stereotype may be reinforced by the fact that only 8.7% of the young adult group had ever sought help for an alcohol problem, and most of the ones who had sought help had attended Twelve Step support groups (e.g., Alcoholics Anonymous) rather than a formal treatment program. One stereotype that was supported by the makeup of this subtype was that it was overwhelmingly male. Only a little more than half of the group worked full-time but over 36% were in school.

The young adult subtype was composed of many binge drinkers as opposed to daily drinkers. They averaged 143 drinking days in the past year but drank more than five drinks (the definition of binge drinking) on nearly three quarters of these drinking days. They were less likely than other subtypes to have co-occurring mental disorders, with a particularly low incidence of Antisocial Personality Disorder. They tended to not have legal problems. This subtype was also characterized by having a family history of alcohol disorders, by cigarette smoking, and by abusing marijuana. They tended to use alcohol in a dangerous manner and to experience alcohol withdrawal symptoms.

FUNCTIONAL SUBTYPE

This group was the third largest (19.4%) and is fascinating because it is not a group that has been widely discussed in the literature on substance use disorders. This may be due to the fact that, despite being older than the other subtypes (average age was nearly 41), only 17% had ever sought help for an alcohol problem. Except for the young adult subtype, this was the lowest percentage of any of the five groups. Furthermore, only about 30% of those who had sought help went to a treatment program, the lowest percentage of any of the groups (they tended to go to Twelve Step groups or private providers such as physicians or mental health professionals). Therefore, treatment providers would have little exposure to the functional subtype and, as was explained earlier, most research has been conducted on treatment populations.

If you are wondering why the group is called "functional," it is because this group (compared to the others) had a remarkable lack of problems. They had the lowest incidence of legal problems, the highest percentage of being married, the second highest rate of full time employment, the second lowest rate of unemployment, and total family income of nearly $10,000 higher than any other group. Over a quarter were college graduates, which was considerably higher than the other groups. Compared to the other subtypes, they tended to have low rates of co-occurring disorders; fewer problems with other drugs; less incidences of alcohol use despite negative consequences; and fewer occurrences of reducing their daily activities as a result of alcohol use (e.g., staying home from work because of a hangover).

The functional subtype had more women than the other groups but it still had nearly 60% males. They began drinking at a later age (18½) and developed alcohol disorders later (around age 37). The members of this group had a fairly high probability of having alcohol disorders in their family history, although most of the other groups were higher. They drank on at least half the days of the year and consumed five or more drinks on more than half of their drinking days. The number of drinking days was the third highest of the groups and the percentage of binge-drinking days was tied for the lowest. They met an average of 3.61 criteria for alcohol dependence, which was the lowest of the five groups but very close to two other groups, including the young adult subtype.

INTERMEDIATE FAMILIAL

This subtype seemed to be a hybrid of the other four groups. Nearly 19% of the people with an alcohol use disorder were in this subtype. As the title of the subtype indicates, there was a relatively high probability that the members had first- or second-degree family members with an alcohol use disorder, although the next two groups we will describe had higher probabilities. The age of onset (32) was the second highest among the groups, as was the age this group started drinking (17). Nearly 64% of this group was male. They had the second highest rate of being married, the second highest rate of being divorced, the second highest percentage of people with a college degree, the second highest family income, and the highest rate of full-time employment (over 2/3). This group was about in the middle with regard to probability of co-occurring disorders and other drug problems.

The intermediate familial group members drank on average about 172 days a year, which was the second lowest among the groups. The number of days they engaged in binge drinking was the lowest (94 days). Almost 27% had at some point sought help for a drinking problem, which was the median of the groups.

YOUNG ANTISOCIAL

This subtype included 21.1% of the people with an alcohol use disorder. As the name implies, they tended to be young (about 26½), to have an early onset of their alcohol use disorder (at about 18½), and to start drinking early (at 15½). Over 3/4 of this group were male, the highest proportion of any of the groups. The individuals in this subtype had the lowest percentage of married members (a little over 15%), the lowest percentage of people with a college degree (about 8%), the second to lowest number who were employed full-time, and were tied for lowest income.

The reason why "antisocial" is in the name of this group is that they had the highest probability of having Antisocial Personality Disorder of any of the subtypes. The topic of Antisocial Personality Disorder will be thoroughly discussed in Chapter 3. At this point, you can get a sense of what this disorder involves by the fact that this group evinced the highest number of antisocial behaviors such as breaking the law, lying, and fighting. They also had high probabilities of having other co-occurring disorders such as major depression, bipolar disorder, and obsessive-compulsive personality disorder. In addition, this group had the highest probability of any of the groups of having marijuana and methamphetamine use disorders and high probabilities of cocaine and opioid use disorders.

The young antisocial group had the second highest number of drinking days (201) per year and the highest percentage (80%) of binge drinking on those drinking days. They also had the largest number of drinks (17) on days they drank alcohol. Consistent with this, this group had the highest probability of having tolerance as a criterion of alcohol dependence.

About 34% of the group (second highest) had ever sought help for a drinking problem. The study did not assess whether subjects had been ordered or "encouraged" to obtain treatment by the criminal justice system. As we will see in Chapter 3, many individuals with Antisocial Personality Disorder only go to treatment when coerced by the criminal justice system.

CHRONIC SEVERE

The most interesting aspect of this subtype is that it is the one most like the "typical" alcoholic but it was the smallest subtype, with only 9.2%. However, nearly 66% of the group had ever sought help for an alcohol problem, which was almost double the next highest group (young antisocial). Over 90% of the people who had sought help had gone to Twelve Step groups and nearly 75% had been in a substance abuse treatment program. Both of these figures are much higher than the other groups. Therefore, although this group has the lowest proportion of people with alcohol use disorders, they are the most likely to be in the most common type of treatment/support settings.

The chronic severe group was about 64% male, with the highest rate of divorce (25%), the lowest family income (effectively tied with the young antisocial group), and the second lowest proportion of college graduates (9%). They had the lowest percentage (43%) of full-time workers.

As might be expected, this group drank the most number of days per year (247), although their rate of binge drinking on drinking days was in the middle at 69%. The largest number of drinks consumed on drinking days was close to the young antisocial group at nearly 15½. They began drinking at about 16 and their age of onset was about 29. They had the highest probability of having family members with an alcohol disorder.

The members of the chronic severe group showed nearly the same number of antisocial behaviors as the young antisocial group. Their probability of having Antisocial Personality Disorder was nearly the same as the young antisocial group. In addition, they had the highest probabilities of having other co-occurring disorders, including major depression, dysthymia, bipolar disorder, generalized anxiety disorder, social phobia, and panic disorder. They also tended to be smokers and to have other substance use disorders. They met the criteria for alcohol abuse more often than the other groups and evinced many of the criteria for alcohol dependence, including withdrawal, persistent efforts to cut down, drinking larger/longer amounts than intended, time spent recovering from alcohol, reduced activities due to drinking, and drinking despite problems.

IMPLICATIONS OF SUBTYPES

The research on subtypes by the scientists of the National Institute on Alcoholism and Alcohol Abuse was the first study to look at the general population rather than patients in alcohol and other drug treatment programs. The results provide insights into some of the reasons why so many people with substance use disorders do not enter treatment and why so many people who do enter treatment do not complete it successfully. First, there was a sizeable group (Functional Subtype) who did not appear to have significant life problems as a result of their alcohol use, and in the absence of significant life problems, people are not motivated to seek treatment. Now, this seems to be contradictory because in order to be diagnosed with an alcohol use disorder, there has to be "trouble." So, "significant life problems" has to be defined relative to the other subtypes. The Functional Subtype met the fewest criteria for an alcohol abuse disorder (average of .59) or an alcohol dependence disorder (average of 3.61) of any of the groups. Therefore, since at least one criterion must be met for diagnosis of an alcohol abuse disorder and at least three criteria must be met for an alcohol dependence disorder, the Functional Subtype group members minimally met diagnostic criteria for an alcohol use disorder in many cases. Furthermore, the members of this subtype had fairly high probabilities (although lower than most of the other groups) of endorsing the tolerance and withdrawal criteria. These criteria are certainly serious and are indicative of alcohol dependence but do not directly involve the social, vocational, family, financial, or legal problems that generally motivate a person to seek treatment. Medical consequences of tolerance and withdrawal may not be noticed for many years. So, there is some logic to the fact that the Functional Subtype group had the second lowest rate of seeking treatment of any of the groups.

The Young Adult Subtype had the lowest rate of seeking help and comparable average number of criteria for alcohol abuse and alcohol dependence to the Functional Subtype. The age of this group combined with the relatively low number of criteria evinced may explain why so few members of this group had ever sought help for a drinking problem. It might be expected that the members of the Young Adult Subtype would "evolve" to the Functional Subtype as they age if they do not develop any additional problems or to the Chronic Severe Subtype if they do develop more difficulties. Alternatively, perhaps some modify their drinking or stop altogether as they get older. Regardless, it is not difficult to understand why so few members of this group had ever sought treatment.

Together, the Young Adult and Functional subtypes composed more than half of the individuals with an alcohol use disorder in this study. This would certainly explain why many of the people who have an alcohol use disorder say they don't need treatment. Of course, there are other reasons why people with alcohol use disorders say that they don't need treatment, including denial and fear. However, many of these people may not have experienced a sufficient number of or severity of life problems to motivate them to seek treatment.

The issues of premature treatment termination and multiple treatment episodes can be understood by examining the Young Antisocial and Chronic Severe Subtypes. The individuals in these groups have multiple, severe problems that complicate treatment. Their employment histories were worse, their education level was lower, they had lower incomes, they met more criteria of the alcohol use disorders, they drank more frequently and in larger quantities, and they had a higher frequency of other substance use disorders than the other groups. In addition, these groups had high rates of co-occurring disorders such as mood disorders, anxiety disorders, bipolar disorder, and Antisocial Personality Disorder. These co-occurring mental disorders complicate treatment and, traditionally, alcohol and other drug treatment programs have not been very successful in working with patients with co-occurring mental disorders. This is due to the fact that alcohol and other drug counselors usually do not have the training and licensure requirements to treat other mental disorders and treatment programs, particularly those funded with public dollars, often do not have psychiatrists, psychologists, and other mental health professionals on staff to provide these services. While the Young Adult Antisocial and Chronic Severe subtypes only compose a little over 30% of the total sample of people with alcohol use disorders, the group members were much more likely to have sought treatment than members in the other subtypes. Therefore, the clients in these two subtypes are hard to treat and more likely to drop out of treatment and/or require multiple treatment episodes.

In the following three chapters of this book, we will look more closely at three classifications of addicts. Let me explain the relationship between the five subtypes described here and the following three classifications. The first includes addicts who fit the classic disease model of addiction. These individuals are many of those who are in the Chronic Severe Subtype, as well as some from other subtypes. These "disease model" addicts are the individuals who are most aligned with traditional models of alcohol and other drug treatment. The presence or absence of co-occurring mental disorders is the best explanation for their treatment success or failure.

The next classification is the group with Antisocial Personality Disorder. This includes the Young Antisocial Subtype and many of the Chronic Severe Subtype. Although some of these individuals may share characteristics of the disease model, I will argue that the fact that they have Antisocial Personality Disorder outweighs any other characteristic and will predict treatment failure.

Finally, I will discuss functional addicts. Obviously, this is the Functional Subtype. This is the understudied group of addicts. They don't go to treatment so they remain undetected. This fairly sizeable group explains why so many addicts say they don't need treatment.

You may be wondering how the largest group, the Young Adult Subtype, fits into this classification. As I said previously, this group has relatively few problems and the individuals don't seek treatment often. Because of their age, the members of this subtype will probably evolve in their drinking and either fit in the Functional, Intermediate Familial, or Chronic Severe subtype at some point, assuming that they do not modify their drinking or stop altogether. (There was a very low probability of Antisocial Personality Disorder in this group, so they would unlikely be in the Young Antisocial Group.) Therefore, it would probably be later in life that it could be determined if the Young Adult Subtype group members would fit the disease model or become functional addicts, assuming they continue to drink heavily.

Following a discussion of these three classifications of addicts (disease model, Antisocial Personality Disorder, functional), the implications of these classifications on early intervention and treatment will be explored.

CASE EXAMPLES

The chapters on the disease model of addiction, Antisocial Personality Disorder, and functional addicts include interviews or stories of people who fit in these classifications. These are real people. Although two of the people did not care if personally identifiable information was included in their cases, I decided to maintain the anonymity of all the people as an added layer of "security" to maintain the confidentiality of all the cases. I know all of the individuals personally except for Melinda (disease-model case example) and Henry and Rick (the Antisocial Personality Disorder case examples). Melinda, Henry, and Rick were recruited by a clinician who I know very well and trust completely. This clinician reviewed the written stories submitted by Melinda, Henry, and Rick and attested to the accuracy of the content. I personally conducted the interviews with George, Mark, and Amy. Steve wrote his story. I know George, Mark, Amy, and Steve well enough to determine the veracity of their stories. Steve, Melinda, Henry, and Rick were paid a fee of $100 each for their stories. George, Mark, and Amy refused to accept any payment. There were other Antisocial Personality Disorder and functional case examples who were recruited but declined to participate.

The case examples were not chosen to illustrate average or typical individuals. They were designed to make the discussions in the chapter more concrete by telling the stories of real people. The stories of Steve and Melinda are pretty typical of disease-model addicts. Henry, one of the case examples of an addict with Antisocial Personality Disorder, probably isn't typical. However, he does illustrate that it is possible to have a relatively successful outcome for an addict with Antisocial Personality Disorder. He is not currently incarcerated and, at least according to him, is managing adequately. Rick's story is seen more typically with this kind of addict. It was challenging to find addicts with Antisocial Personality Disorder who were willing to tell their stories, who could be located, and who were not in a correctional facility that made access impossible.

I can't discuss the methods I used to find functional addicts because of the potential that confidential information would be disclosed. It's not possible to say if these three cases are typical or unusual because so little is known about this group. The fact that all three are professionals with college educations and that two have advanced degrees probably means that they are not representative of the functional group. However, the stories clearly illustrate the concept of functional addicts.

Except for one of the cases (Henry), I did very little editing of the interviews or written stories. I thought it would be best to allow the individuals to express themselves in their own way. Henry's written story was constructed without many of the punctuation and sentence-construction conventions readers are accustomed to seeing. After editing his story, I did send it back to him for approval. The only other editing of the interviews or stories was to correct spelling or typographical errors and to delete irrelevant material from the interviews (e.g., someone saying "you know?" repeatedly).

I feel the need to add a final note of caution about case examples. Using real cases can illustrate a point or concept but they do not prove or validate anything. It would be a mistake to generalize from just a couple of cases. This would be particularly dangerous with the functional addict cases. There is simply not enough information about this group to derive any conclusions from these case examples.

TWO

The Disease Model of Addiction

The disease model of addiction has been depicted in the popular media for some time. From films in the 1960s like *Days of Wine and Roses* (starring Jack Lemmon and Lee Remick) and the 1990s and 2000 (e.g., *When a Man Loves a Woman* (Andy Garcia and Meg Ryan), *Leaving Las Vegas* (Nicholas Cage), *28 Days* (Sandra Bullock), popular books (e.g., *A Million Little Pieces*, James Frey),[1] and television (e.g., *Intervention* on the A&E cable network), the general public has been presented with a view of addiction that is based on the disease model. So, most people are familiar with this model, at least with how it is shown or described for dramatic value.

HISTORY AND CHARACTERISTICS

This popular and controversial model of addiction is credited to E. M. Jellinek, who presented a comprehensive disease model of alcoholism.[2] The disease model has become an implicit component of the Alcoholics Anonymous and Narcotics Anonymous programs, as well as a guiding model for many treatment programs.[3] The World Health Organization acknowledged alcoholism as a medical problem in 1951, and the American Medical Association declared in 1956 that alcoholism was a treatable illness. Following Jellinek's work, the American Psychiatric Association began to use the term "disease" to describe alcoholism in 1965, and the American Medical Association followed in 1966.[4] As with many concepts and theoretical models in the addiction field, the disease concept was originally applied to alcoholism and has been generalized to addiction to other drugs.

The disease of addiction is viewed as a primary disease. That is, it exists in and of itself and is not secondary to some other condition. This is in contrast to psychological models in which addictive behavior is seen as secondary to some psychological condition. In Jellinek's own words:[5]

> The aggressions, feelings of guilt, remorse, resentments, withdrawal, etc., which develop in the phases of alcohol addiction, are largely consequences of the excessive drinking . . . these reactions to excessive drinking—which have quite a neurotic appearance—give the impression of an "alcoholic personality," although they are secondary behaviors superimposed over a large variety of personality types.

Jellinek also described the progressive stages of the disease of alcoholism and the symptoms that characterize each stage.[6] The early stage, or prodromal phase, is characterized by an increasing tolerance to alcohol, blackouts, sneaking and gulping drinks, and guilt feelings about drinking and related behaviors. The next stage, the middle, or crucial, phase, is defined by a loss of control over drinking, personality changes, a loss of friends and jobs, and a preoccupation with protecting the supply of alcohol. The issue of "loss of control" has come to be a central defining characteristic of alcoholism and one of the more controversial aspects of the disease concept. The late stage, or chronic phase, is characterized by morning drinking, violations of ethical standards, tremors, and hallucinations. It is important to conceptualize these stages as progressive. In other words, the stages proceed in sequence and, in the disease model of addiction, are not reversible. Therefore, an individual does not go from the middle stage back to the early stage of alcoholism. The rate at which this progression occurs depends upon factors such as age, drug of choice, gender, and physiological predisposition.[7] For example, adolescents progress more rapidly than adults, females faster than males, and users of stimulants more quickly than alcohol users.[8] Proponents of the disease concept also do not believe that the progression of the disease is affected by a period of sobriety, no matter how long the period of sobriety lasts. As David Ohlms, a physician, has stated:[9]

> let's say that Jack or Jane stops drinking. Maybe because of some formal treatment: maybe he or she just goes on the wagon, and there is a prolonged period of sobriety for, say, 10 or 15 or even 25 years

... then for some reason, ... Jack or Jane decides that they can drink again, and tries to return to the normal, social, controlled type of drinking that any non-alcoholic can get away with. But poor alcoholic Jack or Jane can't. Within a short period of time, usually within 30 days, the symptoms that the alcoholic will show are the same symptoms showed when drinking was stopped 25 years before. And usually worse. It's as if the alcoholic hadn't had that 25 years of sobriety, as if they meant nothing. An alcoholic cannot stay sober for awhile and then start over and have early symptoms of alcoholism.

Consistent with this concept—that the individual with the disease of addiction does not reverse the progression of the disease even with a prolonged period of sobriety—is the notion that addiction is chronic and incurable. That is, if an individual has this disease, it never goes away, and there is no drug or other treatment method that will allow the alcoholic or addict to use again without the danger of a return to problematic use. One implication of this notion is that the only justifiable goal for the alcoholic or addict is abstinence, which is the stance of Alcoholics Anonymous.[10, 11] Furthermore, the idea that addiction is chronic and incurable is the underlying rationale for alcoholics and addicts who are maintaining sobriety for referring to themselves as "recovering" as opposed to "recovered" or "cured."[12]

In addition to the idea that abstinence must be the goal for those with the disease of addiction, there are other implications to the disease concept. First, if the disease is progressive, chronic, and incurable, then it is logical to assume that a person with this condition who does not enter "recovery" will eventually die. Addiction-related deaths usually occur as a result of accidents or the physical effects of alcohol and other drugs over time. However, most of these deaths are not classified as resulting from addiction. For example, in 1994, a member of the Houston Oiler professional football team was involved in a traffic accident in which his best friend was thrown from the car and killed. The football player was so distraught at the sight of his dead friend that he took a shotgun from his car and killed himself. Both men were well over the legal limit for blood alcohol level. The football player's friend had a blood alcohol level over three times the legal limit. These deaths were not classified as the result of alcohol use but as a result of a traffic accident and a suicide. However, a proponent of the disease concept would attribute these deaths to alcoholism. Similarly, consider the individual who, after many years of heavy drinking, develops a liver disease. Eventually, he dies of liver failure.

Is the cause of death liver failure or alcoholism? Again, in the disease concept of addiction, these deaths are the result of untreated addiction.

A further implication of the disease concept of addiction is that, if a person has this disease and, for example, the drug of choice of the person is alcohol, the person will continue to exhibit all the same symptoms of the disease if he or she discontinues the use of alcohol and begins to use some other drug. This is true no matter what the drug of choice is. As long-time addiction educator James Royce stated,[13] "We mentioned the recovered alcoholics who relapse when given a painkiller by the dentist and have seen long-recovered alcoholics whose doctor prescribed tranquilizers after a mild heart attack relapse into alcoholic drinking within three weeks and death in six months." This phenomenon is not restricted to alcohol. "Based on extensive clinical experience, use of any psychoactive drug will usually lead back to use of the primary drug or addiction to the secondary drug (drug switching). I believe the only safe path to follow is complete abstinence from all psychoactive drugs."[14]

EVIDENCE TO SUPPORT THE DISEASE CONCEPT

The evidence to support the disease concept is based on the similarity of alcoholism and drug addiction to other chronic diseases and on research on the brain chemistry and brain changes in addicts. Researchers A. Thomas McLellan, David Lewis, Charles O'Brien, and Herbert Kleber reviewed the literature on chronic illnesses, such as diabetes, asthma, and hypertension, and compared the characteristics of these diseases to addiction. They found that the genetic heritability, established by examining rates of diseases in identical versus fraternal twins, was very similar for alcoholism and drug addiction compared to the other chronic illnesses. In addition, response to treatment is similar. Left untreated, the condition of most alcoholics and drug addicts becomes worse. Remission is unusual. This also occurs with diabetes, asthma, and hypertension.[15] McLellan and his colleagues also showed that the percentages of clients who comply with treatment and the relapse rates of addiction and other chronic illnesses are the same.[16] Addiction, diabetes, asthma, and hypertension are all conditions in which there is no "cure." However, all these problems can be managed through proper treatment, and this treatment must be followed for life. McLellan and colleagues also discussed the issue of the "voluntary" nature of alcohol and other drug use.[17] Again, they compare the choice to use alcohol and other drugs to other chronic illnesses. For example, diet, physical activity, and stress level are all factors affecting hypertension. These factors are all within voluntary control. However, what is not in voluntary control is the person's physiological response to these factors, and the physiological response is strongly influenced by genetic factors. Therefore, addiction is similar to other chronic diseases in that the management of the condition requires voluntary treatment compliance. However, the development of the disease is not due to choice, but to factors beyond voluntary control.

CRITICS OF THE DISEASE CONCEPT

The disease concept is controversial and not without its critics. Probably, the two most famous critics are Stanton Peele and Herbert Fingarette, both of whom have written books[18, 19] as well as articles disputing the disease concept of addiction. Some of their arguments will be summarized here. Since the disease concept is widely attributed to Jellinek, much of the criticism has been directed at his research, which was the basis for his conclusions about the disease concept. Jellinek's data were gathered from questionnaires distributed to Alcoholics Anonymous members through its newsletter, *The Grapevine*. Of 158 questionnaires returned, 60 were discarded because members had pooled and averaged their responses. Also, no questionnaires from women were used. Jellinek himself acknowledged that his data were limited. Therefore, one might wonder why Jellinek's concept of the disease of alcoholism received such widespread acceptance. One reason is that the disease concept is consistent with the philosophy of Alcoholics Anonymous, which is by far the largest organized group dedicated to help for alcoholics. Second, as Peele noted:

> The disease model has been so profitable and politically successful that it has spread to include problems of eating, child abuse, gambling, shopping, premenstrual tension, compulsive love affairs, and almost every other form of self-destructive behavior. . . . From this perspective, nearly every American can be said to have a disease of addiction.[20]

Furthermore, Fingarette accuses the alcohol industry itself of contributing to the public perception of alcoholism as a disease:

> By acknowledging that a small minority of the drinking population is susceptible to the disease of alcoholism, the industry can implicitly assure consumers that the vast majority of people who drink are *not* at risk. This compromise is far preferable to both the old

temperance commitment to prohibition, which criminalized the entire liquor industry, and to newer approaches that look beyond the small group diagnosable as alcoholics to focus on the much larger group of heavy drinkers who develop serious physical, emotional, and social problems.[21] (italics in original)

The progressive nature of addiction has also been criticized. George Vailant, a proponent of the disease concept, has suggested that there is no inevitable progression of Jellinek's stages of alcoholism:

The first stage is heavy "social" drinking. . . . This stage can continue asymptomatically for a lifetime; or because of a change of circumstances or peer group it can reverse to a more moderate pattern of drinking; or it can "progress" into a pattern of alcohol abuse. . . . At some point in their lives, perhaps 10–15 percent of American men reach this second stage. Perhaps half of such alcohol abusers either return to asymptomatic (controlled) drinking or achieve stable abstinence. In a small number of such cases . . . such alcohol abuse can persist intermittently for decades with minor morbidity and even become milder with time.[22]

Similarly, Royce, in describing the patterns and symptoms of alcoholism, stated, "Even when progression occurs, it does not follow a uniform pattern. The steps may be reversed in order, or some steps may be omitted. Symptoms progress, too; something that was minor in an early stage may appear later in a different form or to a greater degree. . . . Rate of progression varies also."[23] As with Vailant, Royce takes a favorable position toward the concept of addiction as a disease.

As we have seen, some of those with sympathetic views toward the disease model of addiction have recognized that the concept of a rigid and inevitable progression of stages is not consistent with reality in working with individuals with alcohol and other drug problems. However, the issue of "loss of control" has been a more contentious one. As Fingarette stated, loss of control may be "the central premise of the classic disease concept of alcoholism."[24] Certainly, the first step of the Twelve Steps of Alcoholics Anonymous implies this loss of control: "We admitted that we were powerless over alcohol—that our lives had become unmanageable."[25] Several arguments have been advanced to dispute the notion of loss of control. Fingarette pointed out that if alcoholics lack control only after first consuming alcohol, then they should have no difficulty abstaining.[26] Obviously, however, alcoholics do have difficulty abstaining from alcohol. If loss of control exists before the first drink (which would explain the difficulty in abstaining), it implies difficulty in exercising self-control or willpower. Experimental studies have demonstrated that alcoholics can exert control over their drinking but variables such as the amount of effort to get alcohol, the environment in which drinking occurs, the belief about what is being consumed, rewards, and the like influence how much is consumed by an alcoholic.[27, 28] As one example, researchers G. Alan Marlatt, Barbara Demming, and John Reid divided alcoholics into four groups. One group believed that they were taste-testing three brands of a vodka-tonic beverage when they were actually drinking tonic water only. A second group believed that they were taste-testing tonic water only, when they were actually drinking vodka and tonic. The third group was correctly told they were drinking a vodka and tonic beverage, and the fourth group was correctly told they were drinking tonic water only. The results showed that it was the alcoholic's belief about what they were drinking that determined the amount they drank and not the actual alcohol content of the beverage they consumed. The alcoholics who expected tonic and got alcohol drank an almost identical amount to those alcoholics who expected and got tonic. Both of these groups drank considerably less than the groups who expected alcohol, and the alcoholics who received and expected alcohol drank nearly the same amount as those alcoholics who expected alcohol but got tonic.[29] Defenders of the disease concept point out that "experimenters took too literally the idea that one drink always means getting drunk," and that "Many research projects set out to disprove the 'one drink' hypothesis in laboratory or hospital settings so artificial and with criteria so wooden that nobody with real experience in alcoholism could take the results seriously."[30] Loss of control has been modified to mean that the alcoholic or addict cannot predict the situations in which he or she will exercise control and the situations in which he or she will lose control. Therefore, this loss of predictability is thought to define the alcoholic or addict.[31] Fingarette's response is that "This new approach to loss of control so emasculates the concept that it becomes useless in explaining or predicting drinking behavior."[32]

ADVANTAGES OF THE DISEASE CONCEPT

Perhaps the greatest advantage to the articulation that addiction is a disease has been to remove the moral stigma attached to addiction and to replace it with an emphasis on treatment of an illness. We do not punish a person for having a disease; we provide assistance. In a more practical sense, defining addiction as a disease has also resulted in treatment coverage by insurance companies. Using medical terminology to describe addiction has also led to greater interest in scientific research. Few medical scientists would be interested in investigating the physiological correlates of a lack of willpower or a moral deficiency. For the individual who has problems with alcohol or other drugs (and for the family as well), the concept of a disease removes much of the stigma and associated embarrassment, blame, and guilt. You would not feel guilty if you were diagnosed with diabetes and, therefore, a person with addictive disease need not feel guilty for having this disease. People who believe that addiction is due to a lack of willpower or to a moral deficiency may avoid treatment, since the admission of the need for help is an admission that some character flaw exists. Therefore, an acceptance of the disease concept may make it easier for some people to enter treatment. Another advantage of the disease concept is that it is clearly understandable to people and provides an explanatory construct for the differences in their alcohol and other drug-taking behavior compared with others. To reuse the well-worn analogy with diabetes, it is quite clear to the people with diabetes that they cannot use certain foods in the same manner as those who do not have diabetes. If they do, there will be certain predictable consequences. Knowledge about the disease allows the alcoholic or addict to understand that he or she is physiologically different from others. In the same way that it may be unwise for the diabetic to eat a hot fudge sundae (in spite of the fact that friends may do so without consequences), the alcoholic learns that it would be unwise to drink (in spite of the fact that friends may do so without consequences). Finally, the disease concept has a logical treatment objective that follows from its precepts: abstinence. If you have a physiological condition that results in severe consequences when alcohol or other drugs are used, you can avoid these consequences by abstaining from alcohol or other drugs. If you attempt to use moderately, you will eventually lose control, progress through predictable stages, and suffer the consequences. Since most individuals who seek treatment for alcohol or other drug problems have experienced some negative consequences already, this argument can be compelling.

DISADVANTAGES OF THE DISEASE CONCEPT

As the critics of the disease concept have pointed out, the orthodox precepts of the disease concept may not be accurate. There is not an inevitable and completely predictable progression of symptoms and stages nor a consistent loss of control. Therefore, individuals with alcohol or other drug problems who may need some form of intervention or treatment may avoid help since they do not fit the "disease model." For example, I was once told by a substance abuse program counselor about an inquiry from a man whose girlfriend thought he had a drinking problem. Although he drank on a daily basis, his use of alcohol had not progressed in the last few years. When asked if he was having any financial, occupational, legal, or family problems, he said that he was not. Now, certainly, denial may be at work here, but the point is that the intake counselor did not encourage the man to seek help because he did not fit the classic "disease" characteristics and the program in which the counselor works was based on this model. Of course, as we have seen from the discussion in Chapter 1, the man may have been a Functional Subtype but this is not generally something that is acknowledged in traditional treatment programs.

An adherence to the disease model may also result in a purely medical model of treatment:

> While this may have the advantage of motivating physicians to treat the alcoholic in a nonjudgmental way . . . the average American physician is still both reluctant to treat alcoholics and often ignorant about alcoholism. . . . Medical models tend to put the physician in full charge, focus almost exclusively on physical damage, and perpetuate a medical "revolving door" which is more humane than the drunk tank but equally ineffective for long-range treatment. It implies that non-medical persons are unable to treat the illness.[33]

The notion that the disease concept removes responsibility from the alcoholic or addict for his or her behavior is frequently cited as a disadvantage of this model.[34] Since the alcoholic or addict is "powerless" over the disease, inappropriate or even criminal behavior may be attributed to the "disease." Relapse may also be blamed on the disease: "If alcoholics come to view their drinking as the result of a disease or physiological addiction, they may be more likely to assume the passive role of victim whenever they engage in drinking behavior if they see it as symptom of their disease."[35] In other words, if an alcoholic believes the disease concept and the AA slogan "one drink away from a drunk," then a "slip" (return to use) may result in the alcoholic's giving up responsibility for maintaining sobriety and returning to a previous level of use, since the slip is seen as symptomatic of the inevitable loss of control. Proponents of the disease concept counter this argument by saying that the addict is not responsible for the disease but is completely responsible for recovery. In addition, court rulings have rarely allowed a defense of addiction for criminal behavior.[36]

ADDICTION AS A BRAIN DISEASE[37]

Over the past 10 to 15 years, the National Institute on Drug Abuse (NIDA) (a federal agency of the National Institutes of Health, which is a part of the U.S. Department of Health and Human Services) has taken the concept of addiction as a disease and provided a scientific context for this model. This context, supported by funded research, describes addiction as a brain disease. According to a publication from NIDA, "Addiction is defined as a chronic, relapsing brain disease that is characterized by compulsive drug seeking and use, despite harmful consequences. It is considered a brain disease because drugs change the brain—they change its structure and how it works. These brain changes can be long lasting, and can lead to the harmful behaviors seen in people who abuse drugs." NIDA scientists have estimated that 40% to 60% of someone's vulnerability to addiction is due to genetic factors. Of course, the environment has an impact on how this vulnerability is expressed. For example, suppose you have a genetic predisposition for addiction. However, suppose you are also a member of the Mormon faith, which prohibits the use of mind-altering substances, including alcohol and caffeine, and you faithfully adhere to the teachings of the church. Since you never use alcohol and other drugs, you will not have any behavioral expression of the genetic predisposition to addiction. On the other hand, let's say you have a slight genetic predisposition for addiction (i.e., one grandparent was an alcoholic). However, you start using alcohol and other drugs in early adolescence and continue to use these substances regularly throughout your teenage years and early adulthood. According to NIDA researchers, the adolescent brain is still developing and alcohol and other drug abuse disrupts brain functioning in areas critical to motivation, memory, learning, judgment, and behavior control. Therefore, early alcohol and other drug use impacts the developing brain and your slight genetic predisposition results in addiction.

If you think that you are safe because you do not have any family history of addiction that you are aware of, remember that only about half of the genetic vulnerability to addiction is due to genetic factors. There are other environmental factors, such as the presence of co-occurring mental disorders that increase the risk for addiction. Also, the type of drugs that are taken, the age you start using alcohol and other drugs, and the method that drugs are administered are also factors that increase the risk for addiction. For example, regardless of your genetic predisposition, if you smoke cocaine (i.e., crack) on a regular basis, you are very likely to become addicted. If you take opioid drugs (e.g., heroin, methadone, oxycondone) every day, you will probably become addicted to them.

Brain-imaging techniques have allowed NIDA researchers to understand how drugs work. Obviously, this is extremely complex and it is beyond the scope of this book to thoroughly explain the anatomy and neurobiology of all these mechanisms. So, simply stated, drugs affect the brain's reward center through chemicals called neurotransmitters. Neurotransmitters are natural chemicals released by the nerve cells in the brain all of the time. When you use alcohol or most other drugs, there is a "flood" of neurotransmitters released in the brain's reward center. With stimulants like cocaine, neurotransmitters in the reward center remain active for much longer than normal. It is this "flood" of neurotransmitters or the long duration of activity that explains why people experience pleasure (i.e., euphoria) when taking mind-altering drugs. Of course, the reward center is not the only area of the brain affected, so that when people use cocaine, they also get more alert and active. Alcohol slows your reflexes. Human beings are "wired" to repeat pleasurable activities. It helps us survive. We want to have sex because it feels good, but sex is how our species continues. If sexual activity were not pleasurable, we would not engage in it frequently enough to perpetuate our species. We have to eat to live, and so eating is a pleasurable activity. Therefore, because of this evolutionary drive, once the reward center is activated by alcohol and other drugs, we want to repeat the experience.

Human brains are quite adaptable. After a period of time of having the reward center artificially stimulated to produce an excess of neurotransmitters in response to alcohol or most other drugs, the brain stops producing a normal quantity of neurotransmitters naturally. At that point, the drug user needs to use drugs just to feel normal. That is what is called "tolerance." The brain has actually changed as a result of drug use. Fortunately, it appears that most brain changes return to normal after a period of abstinence. Of course, that all depends on how long drug use has continued, which drugs were used, and how drugs are administered.

There are many individual differences in human brains and so people react differently to different drugs. Just like one person may love chocolate and another person may be indifferent to it, some people get extreme pleasure from alcohol and other drugs and some people don't. This can also vary by drug. One person may think marijuana is wonderful but they don't like to drink, and someone else can be the opposite. These individual differences probably have a strong genetic component and explain why some people become addicted to alcohol and other drugs so easily and others do not. It has been hypothesized that the addict's brain has a strong reward experience to alcohol and other drugs. That makes the potential addict continue to seek out this rewarding experience to a greater extent than the person without this strong reward experience.

RELATIONSHIP OF THE DISEASE MODEL TO TWELVE STEP RECOVERY PROGRAMS

People often associate the disease model of addiction with Twelve Step recovery programs like Alcoholics Anonymous (AA) and Narcotics Anonymous (NA). This is not unwarranted, since the "bible" of AA, the *Big Book*, states: "We are convinced to a man that alcoholics of *our type* are in the grip of a progressive illness"[38] (italics added). Notice that 75 years ago even the AA literature recognized that there were different types of alcoholics. The other references to alcoholism as a disease are in the personal stories that make up a large part of the *Big Book*. I have attended many AA meetings and the disease model is the predominant conceptualization of the condition. If you ever read the personal stories of Bill W. and Dr. Bob, the founders of AA, they certainly sound like disease model alcoholics.

However, the AA program (the Twelve Steps and the Twelve Traditions) make no reference to any particular model of addiction. In fact, the third of the Twelve Traditions is "The only requirement for AA membership is a desire to stop drinking."[39] So, a person does not have to subscribe to the disease model of addiction to attend Twelve Step recovery meetings. The AA traditions also preclude the organization from taking any position on controversial issues. The point is that AA (or NA) as organizations do not care about models of addiction or subtypes of addicts. People are accepted into the groups if they have a desire to stop drinking or using drugs, and members are encouraged to adopt the Twelve Steps for their recovery program. Nothing else is relevant. So, although the disease model is certainly the way AA members think of their condition, no one should be dissuaded from attending Twelve Step recovery groups if he or she does not think of addiction as a disease.

RELATIONSHIP OF THE DISEASE MODEL TO SUBTYPES

There is not a clean match between the disease model and the subtypes described in Chapter 1 but, at first glance, the Chronic Severe Subtype would seem to be the closest fit. This group had the highest probability of having a family member with an alcohol disorder, they drank the most number of days, and they were the most likely to go to AA or substance abuse treatment. The high rates of Antisocial Personality Disorder and other co-occurring disorders do not preclude the members of the group from displaying the characteristics of the disease model. The disease model does not exclude co-occurring mental disorders, and, in fact, the research by NIDA shows that people with co-occurring disorders are more likely to develop an addictive disorder. However, the Chronic Severe Subtype was the smallest subtype, comprising only a little more than 9% of the people with an alcohol use disorder. It doesn't seem likely that the most popular and long-standing conceptualization of addiction would only apply to less than 1 out of 10 individuals with a substance use disorder.

Let's look at the other subtypes in relationship to the characteristics of the disease model. It is somewhat difficult to see how the Functional Subtype would fit the disease model. The relative lack of problems (compared to the other subtypes) seems inconsistent with what would be predicted from the disease model progression.

The Young Adult Subtype could certainly be composed of individuals who fit the disease model. It may just be too early (chronologically) to tell. The Young Antisocial Subtype may also have disease model alcoholics. The predominant characteristic of this subtype was antisocial personality disorder (APD) but, as was said, this would not preclude members of that subtype from also fitting the disease model. The Intermediate Familial Subtype seems to be a hybrid with no defining characteristic. Certainly, many of the members of this subtype might fit the disease model. However, they drank, on average, less than half the days of the year and had the lowest number of binge-drinking days of any of the subtypes. That doesn't fit the disease model precisely.

What are we to make of this apparent dissonance? The disease model is the predominant way that treatment providers, federal policy makers, and the general public view addiction. Yet, it is difficult from the subtyping study to see the consistency between the characteristics of the disease model and many of the individuals with alcohol use disorders. Let me propose a resolution.

Let's suppose that the NIDA researchers are correct. There are individual differences in the rewarding experience people have from using alcohol and other drugs. But, the differences are on a continuum rather than a dichotomous addict/nonaddict model. On the extreme end, there are those who experience an extremely rewarding effect that produces an unbelievable craving for more. These are classic disease model addicts. However, as you move from the most extreme rewarding experience to the less extreme on the continuum, you may still see many problems from alcohol and other drug use but not necessarily all of the classic characteristics of the disease model. On top of this, the symptoms would be mediated by other environmental factors such as co-occurring mental disorders. So, a person with a moderately high rewarding experience from mind-altering substances who had a depressive disorder might have as many (or more) symptoms as someone with an extremely high rewarding experience but no co-occurring mental disorder. Or, a person with a moderately high rewarding experience who starts injecting heroin will be just as addicted as someone with a very high rewarding experience who drinks. Perhaps we should describe addiction as a brain *condition* rather than as a brain disease.

IMPLICATIONS FOR SUBSTANCE ABUSE TREATMENT

Although I have presented information that conflicts with the classic disease model of addiction, after many years working in this field, I have absolutely no doubt that there are people who fit this model. I have been in meetings with them, worked with them, and treated them. You will read two case studies at the end of this chapter of disease model addicts. There are people who are nice, friendly, productive, moral individuals who are also addicts. During the time that they are in the throes of their addiction, they often act in ways that are nasty, criminal, immoral, and lazy. Once they start recovery (i.e., are abstinent and attending some kind of support group), they again become nice, friendly, productive, and moral individuals. Like most addiction professionals, I believe that these folks have a chronic condition and it is a joy to see them turn their lives around in the face of that condition.

These classic disease model alcoholics were the types of addicts who were in AA when it started and were the patients in the first treatment programs. Treatment was designed for this type of addict. Most of the early treatment programs (and many of them still today) use what is called the Minnesota Model. This is based on the principles of AA and relies heavily on counselors who are in recovery themselves and may not have any formal counselor training. As treatment populations became more heterogenous (women, adolescents, people with co-occurring disorders, criminal justice populations), treatment became more complex. There have been and continue to be many efforts at the state and federal level to adapt to the diversity and complexity of the treatment population by increasing training and requirements for addiction counselors, discovering and implementing evidence-based treatment practices, and collecting outcome data to measure client progress. However, like any entrenched system, change is resisted and so, change happens slowly. As we have seen, many or most of the addicts in treatment do not fit the classic disease model but the treatment system has been designed for addicts who do.

This may explain, to some degree, why so many people in treatment terminate it before completion and why so many return to treatment over and over again.*

CASE EXAMPLES
Steve's Story

At 17, I drank my first Olympia beer and had my first drunk. I peeled the paper labels off with my thumb, looked at the dots on the back and fantasized about getting lucky at [name of place] in May of my senior year [Author's Note: There was a game with this brand of beer. Each label had one to four dots, perhaps indicating the bottling location. The number of dots indicated how far you would get with your date that night]. The feeling and the people are perpetually bright, even though it was 46 years ago. I felt the great "AHHH!" I was released from the bondage of anxiety and fear. I've always believed I was a powdered alcoholic. The artesian well-water of Olympia, an old marketing term, loosed my alcoholism.

That May evening was the first time I felt comfortable with my friends, even though I had gone from kindergarten through senior high with most of them. I played football, basketball and baseball, and ran track. For the first time I didn't feel like an outcast, I didn't have that low level anxiety, that churning in my guts because I didn't know why I couldn't connect with them and I wanted to.

The next weekend I drank with my "new friends," splitting a six pack. After quickly drinking my two, I felt this strange craving to drink more. I tried to talk them into giving me more. I don't know if they did, I just remember that craving.

My Dad's brother, my one-legged, Uncle A. drank often and smuggled Canadian Club back into the states from Canada. I loved my Uncle. He took me haying, took me with him while he sat sprinkler pipe; took me on trips when he went to buy cattle, let me tend the wood stove at the auction company on sale day. He was all the things I thought I wasn't: competent, confident, assured, at ease in social settings, comfortable and successful. He was a very functional alcoholic. I never thought my Dad

---

*Other explanations will be explored later in this book. With regard to the disease model of addiction, relapse is a common aspect of chronic conditions, so returning to treatment would not be unexpected.

drank much. But people would come to our house after drinking at a bar where he went after work. It was a normal social setting in our small community. Their barbershop singing woke me up. He and Mom belonged to a very social group, called the "Thinking and Drinking Society." I never thought much about it, just a gathering they went to once in a while, and listened to stories about the folks who drank and got silly.

I made home brew, which was poisonous, vinegary and had a huge kick. We drank "store bought" or "home brew."

I went to a small college to play football, no scholarship and got a major injury. My freshman year I was a three-sport varsity lettermen, mostly by default, because one letter was in wrestling. I'd never wrestled before but I weighed 195 pounds, so my coach said I was the heavyweight. I went up against real heavyweights who weighed between 215 and 245 pounds and had wrestled since were infants. One was a Pacific Coast Champion. The match was very short. Canvas back was my nickname.

As a sophomore, I got kneed in the head and got a concussion. Later, I got clipped twice, rupturing two discs, breaking a bone in my ankle and straining knee ligaments. My playing days were over. I had two back surgeries, which provided absolutely no relief.

I gained a scar, but lost my identity as a jock, and the protective exoskeleton of pads, uniforms and the insect helmet. I began to drink weekends and some week nights, while taking Vicodin and Percocet's for the chronic sciatic pain. By 20, I was drinking mostly on weekends, but had horrific hangovers, which would beach me on the couch of the fraternity's TV room. I took 20 aspirins a day for 20 years. The Vicodin didn't provide any relief from the hangovers or maybe I didn't know about taking them. At one semester break, one hangover kept me on the cool tiles of the shower floor while I puked for about 24 hours, and then staggered into my car to drive home.

I puked my entire drinking career. Blackouts and passing out, burning myself with the heating pad I used for the pain, waking up with puke on my T-shirt, puking bile. To stop one puking episode of 12 or 14 hours, I needed a Thorazine suppository to stop. I reconciled that through my Christian upbringing: "The wages of sin."

At 19, I knew I had a drinking problem. A campus visit by some religious organization provided some counseling awareness that I had the problem and could do something about it. I was to see him the next day. Memory fades. Either he didn't come back or I didn't go back. This was a really bleak time.

And I didn't feel very comfortable in class rooms. I never talked. I didn't talk until I was a senior in a small seminar class; even then it was brief and agonizing. I walked around anxious. Writing papers was painful. A chronic sense of less than, inadequacy and a heavy case of social butterflies. Drinking let me feel comfortable, adopt a Falstaffian personae.

Despite my drinking and drugging, I was on the Dean's list, a tutor and graduated, with distinction. Having absolutely no plans for the future, I remember hearing that senior finals were coming up. I had not considered the fact that I would graduate in two months, so I scurried to send out a resume for a teaching job. I taught high school and drank. I taught German, which I had earned a D in, and U.S. History which I had never taken. We never got to the Civil War. My students couldn't read, so reading discussions on the themes, styles and "hidden" meanings in my English classes was frustrating for both of us. So, I started a remedial reading class, one of the most rewarding things I have ever done. Since I knew nothing about remedial reading, I stole ideas, consulted that is, from real reading teachers in the system, convinced my principal to fund it and started. They were great kids.

I courted my first wife in a bar, driving ten miles out to get her while cradling travelers driving back to town, drinking pitchers of beer, and then driving her back to the wheat ranch. The daughter of an alcoholic, she tolerated me and then finally caved to my entreaties, though even now, I think she knew better. I was drunk the night before my wedding; very hung-over the day of it, and drank afterwards while I drove to our honeymoon retreat, killing a dog on the way. I stopped and buried it. The first time she saw me sober and not hung-over was several months after we were married. I drank that marriage up. I was an emotional freight train on a roller coaster track.

While coaching the JV high school wrestling team, I stayed up late drinking before an early morning road trip. I must have been sweating badly, stinking badly and driving badly. I was reported and my principal, a wonderful WWII aircraft-carrier pilot, wanted to know if I had been drinking. I denied it, blaming my problems on my insulin-dependent diabetes, a wonderful scapegoat for all my ills.

Despite having fun and success teaching high school, I wanted a master's degree. After my injuries, as an undergraduate, I was a student coach for receivers and line-backers for my little college team. When I wanted to go graduate school, I contacted my former coach who got me a graduate assistantship in football while I was admitted to the master's program in English. I coached, graded film, taught activity classes, while studying Beowulf, Chaucer, Faulkner, etc. I continued to drink, have dreadful hangovers and survive. My marriage didn't. I got my master's, taking my orals in a rolling blackout, saying, as best I can recall, "I don't know" a lot. I worked for the university and got a job in administration. I'd been a summer hire and my boss liked me. He wanted to hire me full time and so wrote a job description for a new position which asked for a journalism degree. While working for him, I went back to school, got my Journalism degree and had more rolling blackouts while taking classes. I believe I asked the same question in the same class, two or three weeks running.

Naturally, I found another alcoholic's daughter. She had the good fortune of leaving the city before our relationship culminated in something really ugly, like marriage. I drank Tequila and gin with her casino-connected father, Pouilley-Fuisse with the family at dinner, and more booze, later, by myself. At casino shows, I drank outrageously.

I worked every day. I would come to the office and puke in the wastepaper basket. Because I became seriously fatigued, my GP hospitalized me. After tests were run, he said I had "metabolic hepatitis." If drinking or booze was discussed, I don't remember it. My diabetes was compromised.

After my girlfriend left, I found an alcoholic woman. We had a tumultuous courtship, so, naturally we decided to marry. That was the beginning of the dark years, not because of the problems in the relationships but because the curtain came down on my memory. The vaults are dark for the last three or four years of my drinking and the first two or three years of sobriety. I operated in blackouts. I came to from a blackout and found myself talking. Friends told me that during these times they'd schedule something with me; I'd agree but never show up.

I bought a direct mail marketing business and left the university. I worked long hours, fought with the post office and became the "dean of direct marketing." But, ultimately, I didn't have any business sense, even though I understood the principles of direct marketing. I'd quit work around 10:00 pm, buy two, 24 ounce beers at the convenience store and finish one in the 10 minutes on the drive home. I'd stash that one, open the other, finish it, then start on the Stolichnaya because I'd been reading Joseph Wambaugh and that's what his protagonists drank. I was soon sloshed and staggered to bed. I'd start the day over. Sometimes puking, sometimes not. I spent at least four years on this treadmill.

One time at work, I shit blood. I rationalized that the blackish, reddish stool was the result of eating beets. I hadn't eaten beets in 10 years. Both the second marriage and the business were in the toilet. Somewhere in October or November of 1980, having stayed in bed for several days, probably from depression and the effects of drinking, I flew to [name of city] to see my folks. While there, I cried spontaneously. I asked my Dad to pray for me. We went to his church, knelt in a middle pew and he prayed aloud for me, with no clue about my problem. I bawled until snot flew; I could not stop crying. Poor Dad. He had two crazy kids; me with my drinking and my bipolar sister. I didn't stop drinking then, but would within four months.

My second wife and I fought. I flew into rages. Once when I felt particularly put upon, I took a five-iron and, starting from about a foot off the floor, knocked holes all the way up to waist-high. I ripped a tie in half while it was on my neck. I hid from friends. I finally moved out when she didn't put toilet paper back on the toilet paper roll. That's right. I couldn't live with someone that irresponsible! I lived in a motel and for dinner I ate a banana, three or four Oreos and two or three, 24-ounce beers. The banana was for my health; a token nod to my diabetes.

The night of my last drunk, I knew I was going to get drunk. I drove to a friend's house so he would drive me to a tour of a local print shop. The tour took about 20 minutes. To prepare for the adventure, I put a beer in each pocket of my sport jacket, took one in each hand and was ready. My friend drove me home. I got in my car. His son came over and asked me how I was doing? I mumbled, "Oogah, aww, ssowhich, uh." Something like that. He looked very surprised and walked away. I was too drunk to talk or walk, but I could drive.

At that moment, I told myself, "You have a drinking problem. You're going to call AA, go to meetings and get sober. And you're life is going to get better." That was in the early morning hours of March 6, 1981. A moment of clarity. I haven't drunk since.

I moved in with a friend who had an extra room. The divorce dragged on and on. I'd quit drinking, but I wasn't sober. During the counseling, cum-reconciliation, sessions I'd become enraged, and say, "It's not you or the topic, it's my head." And I knew it was my alcohol and drug addled mind. AA says, "Your mind is out to kill you." It was.

My friend kept the remnants of a case of beer in his refrigerator left over from his New Year's Eve Party. It didn't bother me. Each morning I packed a lunch, put it on the counter and went to work. Each evening, I'd return, take the brown sack off the counter and put it back in the refrigerator. I threw out the lunch after a week of doing this. I couldn't remember anything.

I went to a meeting a day for five years and found myself in AA. I met Paul, who refused to be my sponsor, but answered my desperate calls on Sunday afternoons. "You've got the Sunday afternoon boarding house blues, huh?" We'd talk. He'd end with, "They closed every meeting in Des Moines (Iowa, far, far away) last night and didn't talk about your problems once." He helped me look at my self-centeredness.

I knew about AA meetings. I called Central Office. When Mary D answered, I asked "Do you have any meetings?" Pretty clever, huh? The

Dean's list guy with a Master in English was a basket case. Mary D said of course and there was one tonight. For whatever reason, I had things to do and couldn't possible go tonight! But within a few days, I drove to the Alano Club, parking several blocks away so I wouldn't be recognized. I walked into the club with a black jacket and pants, shaking, and listened glumly to the laughter, feeling out-of-place. The meeting started; the chairperson, who would later die from her disease, asked for newcomers. I said, "Hi. My name's Steve, and I'm an alcoholic." The great weight was lifted, my secret was out and I felt relieved.

At my first meeting, an Eskimo appeared, John F. He's not a real Eskimo. It's a term AA uses to describe the active presence of God in our lives, manifested by people, leading us out of life's Arctic snow storms when we're about to die, described by a drunk who said God didn't help him escape his storm, "it was some goddamn Eskimo."

John asked me what I was doing the next night. I looked at him blankly. I couldn't think that far ahead. He said he'd pick me up and take me to meetings. We went to meetings and coffee and company afterwards. But I was so tired, I couldn't stay out late and told him, "I'll go with you to meetings, but I'm not going for any goddam coffee afterwards." Always the grateful newcomer. I went to bed early believing that if I stayed up past 11:00 I'd be drunk!

I liked AA from the start. I felt at home, awkward, at first, but at home, accepted. The love and acceptance was palpable. I was very sick physically, mentally and emotionally. My grey pallor, stooped posture, and shakes suggested to a nurse that I had about a couple of weeks left to live had I continued to drink. I shook for the whole month of March. I decided the pain pills were probably not helpful, so I stopped them, abruptly. I had stomach cramps. I couldn't sleep. I couldn't talk without crying. If someone asked how I was, I cried. I couldn't remember simple words, like: cup, glass, sugar, paper or pencil. People finished my sentences. I couldn't remember anything I read or heard. I ached with loneliness. I suffered from "terminal loneliness": it was only marginally better in early sobriety.

I just knew that in the halls of AA, great wisdom sailed all around me and into me and that I was in the presence of something mysterious and wonderful. I tried to capture it in notebooks and on the margins of my AA book. And prayed.

At my first meeting, I got a Big Book and was told to read Chapter 5. When I got home I opened it and looked for Chapter 5. I couldn't find it. Since I had started a reading class and knew about book construction and read all those books, I knew there was a "thing-a-ma-jig" in the front (Table of Contents!). I couldn't find that either. I knew that I'd gotten the only Big Book with neither Chapter 5 nor a table of contents. Rationalization is a killer.

Since March 6, 1981, I've learned that all storms pass, that this too shall pass. I remarried, for the third time, but it's my first sober marriage. I got another degree, my first sober one. I can write more easily. My wife, step-kids and grandkids love me. They kept a vigil in the hospital while I lay dying from infection following a six-way bypass. When my doctor and fellow member of AA told them I was likely to die, they came to my bed, one-by-one to tell me they loved me and thank me for being in their lives.

Four years later, I'm still in their lives and the quality of my life is so much better. Keep coming back.

Analysis of Steve

It isn't necessary to spend much time looking at the diagnostic criteria for substance use disorders we discussed in Chapter 1. Steve clearly had an alcohol dependence disorder. He met every criterion.

Steve's story is a very typical disease model addict story that you would be likely to hear if you went to a meeting of Alcoholics Anonymous. There are a couple of aspects to his story that make his case interesting, although nearly all the stories you hear in AA are quite compelling. Steve discusses his frequent vomiting from heavy alcohol use. If you have ever gotten sick from drinking too much, you know how extremely unpleasant the experience is and how rotten you feel the next day. Despite having this extreme negative reaction to alcohol over and over again, Steve kept drinking. One has to be impressed with the strength of the urge to drink that must be present to override the negative consequences of alcohol. Steve also tells us of the immediate gratification he experienced the first time he drank. He does not talk about having to develop a "taste" for alcohol they way most people do when they begin to drink. Many disease model addicts tell a similar story. Not only did alcohol relieve his anxiety and make him more comfortable socially, he also rapidly experienced the need for more. Again, it is very typical to find that disease model addicts have a much more positive experience with alcohol and other drugs than others do and that they have this strong reinforcement the first time or shortly after the first time they start to drink or use drugs.

Steve's type 1 diabetes is a factor that makes his case a model for the power of addiction. It is not advisable for diabetics to drink heavily. Without going into too much detail, moderate alcohol use raises blood sugar but heavy alcohol use can lower blood sugar to dangerous levels. Alcohol interferes with oral diabetes medicines and insulin. It increases triglyceride levels and blood pressure. Alcohol has a lot of calories. Heavy alcohol use over a long period of time has a damaging effect on every system in the human body. Clearly, it can't be good for a diabetic (or anyone for that matter) to drink the way Steve describes. However, Steve was aware of his diabetic condition, treated himself with insulin, and was well educated. In spite of this, he drank very heavily. The seventh criteria for a substance dependence disorder (see Chapter 1) says that "the substance use is continued despite knowledge of having a persistent or recurrent physical or psychological problem that is likely to have been caused or exacerbated by the substance. . . ." That was Steve, and it illustrates how, for a disease model addict, nothing is more important than the drug of choice.

Steve doesn't tell us a tremendous amount about his family history, but the little he does relate is not the typical story one usually hears from disease model addicts. It sounds like an uncle was a heavy drinker (perhaps a functional addict, as we will discuss in Chapter 4) but, while his parents drank, he doesn't describe them as alcoholics. Nor does Steve describe an abusive or neglectful family history. Although this does not rule out a genetic component to Steve's alcoholism (i.e., we do not know about his grandparents), it does say something about disease model addicts. It is typical to hear stories of horrendous childhoods among disease model addicts since; in many cases, primary caretakers were also addicts. However, it is also not unusual to have disease model addicts describe very normal, loving childhoods. This raises the suspicion that there is just something different (genetically or physiologically) between disease model addicts and nonaddicts.

Steve's story is also unusual in the manner in which he began his recovery and the course of his recovery. It seems strange that with all the terrible experiences he had as a result of his drinking—the failed marriages, blackouts, vomiting, business problems, cognitive difficulties, and violent outbursts—what finally provided the impetus for Steve to stop drinking was his inability to be articulate with a friend's son. I'm not doubting Steve's accuracy or sincerity. After many years of hearing stories from disease model addicts, you never know what event is going to be the one that initiates recovery. Once Steve went to his first AA meeting, it was analogous to his first experience with alcohol. He knew he was in a place that was right for him.

What is unusual about Steve's story is that, considering his long history of alcohol abuse, his medical condition, and his problems in his life, he never went to formal treatment nor did he ever have a slip or relapse since his initial decision to stop drinking. That is quite uncommon, but it is an example of the diversity of paths to recovery.

Melinda's Story

I am a member of the CIA: Catholic Irish Alcoholic. I learned of this elite club in Alcoholics Anonymous; I learned many things in Alcoholics Anonymous, among them, that I am an alcoholic. In the beginning when I was introduced to AA, I did not feel I was like other members and could not relate to the stories or testimonials of recovery. I was happy that these folks had found an answer, but I did not suspect that I had a problem. Even after my first rehab and my first DUI, I felt I was more a victim of exhaustion, misunderstanding and bad luck than I was an alcoholic.

My strict upbringing, my years of controlled drinking and my place in society confirmed that theory. I would simply try harder, be more careful and not work so much thus avoiding the situations that were causing my problems. My rational mind had a field day with these theories and my well meaning family, friends and therapists supported this conclusion. At the time of these events, around the early 1990s, I had experienced lots of stressful situations which anyone would have probably drunk over. It was just 1986 that at age 29 I had been diagnosed with breast cancer. Up till that point, I was living the ideal life of a woman born in 1956. The oldest of seven born to two college educated parents, I was the first woman student body president of my high school. I excelled in nursing school, traveled over the world with my adventurous husband and birthed two sons in 1982 and 1984. Cancer shattered my world. Chemotherapy and reconstruction followed along with the determination to carry on as if everything was fine. I threw myself into service for cancer survivors, reaching out both in education and visiting new patients. I won several awards for these efforts and was county president of the American Cancer Society and seated on the state Board of Directors. I returned to nursing, first as an oncology nurse, then as a hospice nurse and later care coordinator for the area hospice patients. I co-authored a book chapter on pain management and lectured on cancer, hospice and pain management in the area and around the country for the American Academy of Pain Management.

Meanwhile, back home my husband and I came into a large sum of money and invested in a helicopter company; within two years we lost most of it. He sank into a depression and I became more determined than ever to save the family and save the day. I was thirty-three years old. My ego was charged and my life was fueled by self will. I discovered that a glass of wine or two would take the edge off of a tough day, then maybe a little more wine. Everyone around me was drinking about the same so it never occurred to me that this was problematic. My husband and

I discovered fancy drinks that worked well with entertaining and seemed to be popular with our crowd. Soon, having a couple of drinks before the guests was routine, Sunday morning brunch allowed for alcohol to be fashionably served. We only ate at restaurants that served alcohol. He drank as much as I so again, my measuring stick and rational mind didn't suspect anything unusual. He eventually started to volunteer at our sons' school and went on to become a teacher. We found ourselves running successful parallel lives with less and less intersecting. Eventually we found other members of the opposite sex to comfort us. I felt my life was manageable, not perfect, but manageable.

Suddenly, the line was crossed, I didn't see it coming. My parents, sister-in-law and best friend did an intervention and I surrendered to a rehab hospital for 21 days. Unfortunately, they left my husband and my employer out of the information loop. I lost my job (who simply felt I went to lunch and then no call no show for a week as I was not allowed phone calls for my first week of inpatient). My husband was livid, blaming me for this mess (the intervention crew wanted to get him next!). In rehab, I discovered people whose lives were way out of control. Man, they needed this! Not me. When the director of the hospital lost his son to a hang gliding accident, I found myself in the role of grief counselor and with my hospice background and "I'm fine" attitude, set about to be discharged. I was just in need of a little R&R. My work eventually took me back as a per diem home health nurse, my husband forgave me and blamed the interveners and I went to graduate school. The manageability was back in full force and I returned, resolving to try harder and to be smarter.

Eventually, my husband and I realized our marriage was over, but a year of bitter dispute followed. Armed with my hospitalization, he threatened to have me declared an unfit mother. I gave up the fight and lost many things including my sons residing with me. They moved to [name of state] with him. After a couple of months, we smoothed things out, and they have been right since. That is its own story. All through this my drinking was moderated. Maybe it wasn't so bad after all.

I began to mourn the many losses in my life and became determined to pick up the pieces. I had been to [name of state] many times and often wished to live there. Now was a perfect opportunity. I found a man who wanted to be a dive master. A former Navy seal, he took my drinking in stride and with my money and ambition, we set out to live in [name of state]. I found a home in [name of place], talked to the hospital about working there and was determined to show the world once again that I was fine. I was drinking a lot. It was 1994 and I wasn't so sure about this man. I realized I had thrown myself into a dream that had no depth and no soul. I was suffering from a soul sickness that no move would cure. Even as much as my heart and soul had always cried out for paradise, I knew this was empty.

I had heard that one of my hospice families had lost another member; I called to offer my condolences and my help with the services. An old family friend answered the phone. We met at the funeral and reunited. I said good bye to the Seal and [name of state] and hello to my salvation. Here was want I longed for: family! He had two daughters the same ages as my sons. We reminisced and chatted about the familiar. I was drinking more and more, not hiding it for it seemed okay, for awhile. Then, I couldn't control it all the time. More than once, I drank too much or too soon or more than I wanted to drink. I hid alcohol; I didn't want him to know how much I drank. He had put me on a pedestal. The girls thought I was their fairy godmother.

Then, the worst thing ever shattered my world: DUI

Now everyone would know! I was not in control and my life was in ruins. It was April of 1995. This beautiful man knew if he just loved me enough, I'd get better; he knew it was a disease. That's it, it's just a disease and if I don't drink and do everything the court orders, we'll be fine. So we got married and blended these families. Everyone was happy, especially me. I had my four children, my husband, my beautiful house and I had a new job and we were going to live the dream. I threw myself into being the supermom I knew I could be. Along the way I dropped in at a few AA meetings, and threw myself into a spiritual way of life. I worked in alternative medicine and became a healing touch reiki master. I walked a spiritual path. I used AA for social connections and after DUI School, became versed in the way of alcohol. My spiritual path and my family would be all I needed. And it was for three years.

The inconveniences of raising four teenagers and working full time seemed to become more annoying. My husband was controlling where once he had been thoughtful, penny pinching where once he had been frugal. My work was tedious where once it had been stable. People, places and things were not cooperating with my outlook on life. Where once I had blessed situations, I grew annoyed and where once my heart was full of compassion for others, people's drama left me bitter. I was restless, irritable and discontent. My mom was diagnosed with breast cancer in August 1998; I felt my world crashed and I could not figure out why. I reached out to others and found no empathy. On top of that, I was accused of drinking on the job. My alcoholic behavior didn't need any alcohol to emerge. No program, no spiritual path and loneliness, self pity and defeat set in. I was fired from my job and then reported to the state board of nursing who told me to surrender my license. What the hell happened? My friend John Barleycorn welcomed me into the insanity once more. It was 1999 and I struggled to make sense of it all. I would drink and be dry, weeks on and weeks off. I sought help from a psychiatrist who diagnosed me as bipolar. Medication dosages were adjusted every month; now I really felt nuts.

My husband and I worked together to find a solution. Our friend in [name of state] told us of a treatment center in [name of city], [name of treatment program]. In September of 2000, I entered inpatient care. I loved it! I felt the strength to admit to my disease; I was treated by caring professionals and thrived. I missed my family but we all knew this was the solution. And it was, until I had to come home: home to the same people, places and things, home to no aftercare or program of recovery and home to a disease that patiently waits for you. My husband insisted I had the problem and if only I quit drinking, everyone would be better. He refused counseling or Al-anon. I went to AA meetings, but they seemed more social. Even my sponsor felt we were too friendly to keep me sober. So I set out on a spiritual path, after all, in the '90s that approached worked so well. So I did okay and scheduled a retreat to [name] monastery to retreat into my spiritual self. Driving to [name of place] in October 2001, I stopped to buy some lunch and a few club cocktails and individual bottles of wine, just to relax when I arrived. I got lost about a mile from the retreat center; frustrated, I pulled over to a farm house, proceeded to drink and went to the house to ask for directions. The people called the police and I was arrested for DUI.

What an ordeal. This wasn't working. Hospitals, jails and institutions and no solution could be found. It was time to get real. February 2, 2002 I quit the bipolar medication (I wasn't getting better!), I divorced my husband, and the kids went on to college. I went to AA and met up with a life coach who I had done some alternative workshops [with] (breathwork). I was on my way! I became a biosync consultant, learning bodywork that treated a person holistically and lived a physical program of eating mostly raw food, walking and qi gong and aikido, a mental program of studying anatomy and physiology and a spiritual program filled with Buddhist principles and Carolyn Myss. I didn't feel ready to work as a body worker, but discovered I could teach anatomy and physiology to students. This was great. Teaching gave me the space to flex my professional yearnings, nurture staff and students and live my spiritual life. Quietly and humbly, I did just that. Soon came the promotions and recognitions. I developed programs, doubled the student population and became the Medical Department chairman.

At this time, I had met up with another alcoholic in early recovery, someone I had acquaintance with since my youth. Once again, the familiar stepped in: he knew my family and his knew me, he lived on the street where I had raised my young sons and he had three sons: family! Bingo! We moved in together. Wasn't long when he took away my pedestal; no matter, I would be fine without his tenderness. Then, he started drinking; no matter, I was sober. So once again, I threw myself into my professional life rising to the top. We parted in December of 2005 suddenly. It was Christmas and I needed some place to live.

I found solutions, reunited with my children, worked harder, kept fit spiritually, mentally and physically, and stayed sober. I enjoyed my students, but was feeling unappreciated by my coworkers and administration. I was lonely and sad. I isolated more, tried online dating, and felt increasingly depressed. I had been sober for five years. I don't remember picking up that first beer, but I do remember that the voice said vodka would take me there faster. Didn't it used too? I showed up for work one morning having had a beer, admitted to drinking to the president and director of education, told them I was an alcoholic. We agreed that since I had seven weeks of paid time off coming to me, that a five week outpatient program would be just what I need. Of course, a little R&R for the exhaustion, reacquainting with my sobriety principles and I'd be just fine. And they reassured me that no one at work would know my little secret. When I returned to work, everyone knew, and what's more—wouldn't I address addiction with the 300 students by telling my story? Fortunately, my counselors and I convinced them that this was a bad idea. But six months later when I was accused of drinking on the job, I quit. This nightmare was over.

I decided to go into business for myself incorporating Biosync; healing touch and reiki into a practice I called Inspired Life. I hung out my shingle and set up a website and rented an office space. Business was slow, but my clients were enthusiastic about the work. I spent more time at home, marketing on the internet and making calls. Over the past five years I had developed a friendship with a couple; I had worked with him teaching. We would walk for exercise several times a week. Early in 2008, I became increasingly too tired to walk, experiencing respiratory difficulties and general malaise. By April, I could hardly walk and my thinking was fuzzy. This couple took me into their home to assist me in recovery from the mysterious change in health. While we were moving me out of my little rental, we discovered toxic mold as the culprit with moss growing along the roof line as the indicator of bigger problems. R&R renewed my physical health but I was depressed. No home, no income and no job, I was steeped in self pity, fear and despair. I drank.

Within a few weeks, I drank around the clock, never able to capture any control and not wanting to. I kept a supply next to my bed. One morning, I ran out and the driving to restore my supply landed me in a rollover and a resulting DUI.

July 7, 2008 is my sobriety date. I returned to AA meetings humbly announcing as a newcomer. I took a secretary service commitment and found a sponsor. All the while, my roommates stood by me—as long as I was sober. I did the court ordered counseling, alcohol testing and driving breathalyzer. I spoke to nurses in recovery and contacted the state board of nursing to look into the possibility of reinstating my license. I began a weekly nurse support group, saw my sponsor weekly and began to work the twelve steps of Alcoholics Anonymous. I was sober and discovered a new hope. I started a job at a warehouse doing data entry, today I am the Office Supervisor. Slowly working the steps I saw where my chief character defect of pride and its clever disguises of shame, doubt and image preserving had been my undoing. Persons, places and things were given their control back; I was no longer in charge.

Working step one, I accepted that I was powerless and that this disease had been trying to kill me. I fell into my higher power's loving embrace in step two; catching the signs and symbols He left in my path to remind me of His power, love and guidance. I knelt with my sponsor to say the third step prayer and felt the bliss of surrender to His will. I read Harry Tiebout and discovered the difference between compliance and surrender. I understood compliance; I had been compliant all my life. I did not understand how compliance kept me from absolute surrender. The readings turned on the light and one aha moment followed another. I began a book study with about eight other alcoholics and we spent four weeks discussing "The Hound of Heaven." I was able to use recovery literature to keep me academically engaged and mentally excited about my recovery.

My reinstating my license continued at the same pace. The Board would throw me a curve ball or task to accomplish parallel to the step I was working. By the time I had listed my character defects and did a fifth step, my application and theory education was completed. The steps continued and I embraced each one fueled by the grace that I gained with each step. The graces had names like honesty, hope, faith, courage, integrity, willingness, humility, love, justice/discipline, perseverance, awareness and service and discovered these were the principles of the program. These were the principles of each step. Steps eight and nine added more miracles as amends were lovingly given and received. I have a beautiful relationship with my parents and my children not only restored but deeper and richer as well.

Soon ten, eleven and twelve found their way into my life where they live today. I went to an eleventh step retreat and committed to a meditation practice. At this time I began working with a sponsee and found the ultimate in service: giving back what I had so generously had been given. Today, I have a ritual that keeps me sober. As someone pointed out the word ritual is found in spiritual. I awake with God as my first breath and the third, seventh and eleventh step prayers follow. I jump out of bed eager to bring my principles to whatever life serves up. I practice and it's not perfect, but it is from the heart. I speak softer and it is the language of the heart. I find I have more compassion and less judgment, more love and tolerance and less anger and fear. My higher power walks with me throughout the day and His three angels whom I've named Gratitude, Acceptance and Surrender gently but firmly guide my steps.

Today, I went to [name of city] to meet with the [name of state] State Board of Nursing and was given reinstatement of my RN license. It took two years of intense work and perseverance with many generous people giving their love and support. I begin a five year contract after I complete the clinical refresher course. All I know is that I will do it one day at a time. I have many stories of daily miracles that demonstrate the power of the AA recovery if one fully surrenders to God; I suspect I will enjoy many more. My formula for a quiet mind and peace of heart is staying in the now. Bill W. called emotional sobriety the next frontier; I'm ready!

Analysis of Melinda

As has Steve, Melinda has suffered from an alcohol dependence disorder for many years. While her story does not document any withdrawal symptoms, she describes tolerance (increasing her alcohol use to achieve the desired effect), inability to control her alcohol use, repeated DUIs, hiding alcohol, drinking on the job, unsuccessful treatment episodes, and other consequences resulting from her alcohol use. Because of the way Melinda constructed her story, it is difficult to document all the necessary criteria in terms of a 12-month period for diagnostic purposes, but the severity of her problem is clear.

What is striking about Melinda's story is her repeated relapses. As you recall, Steve never had a slip or a relapse after making the commitment to attend AA. He never went to a formal treatment program in spite of having very significant health issues as a result of his drinking. Melinda reports that she entered treatment after an intervention from family members, went to a psychiatrist, enrolled in another treatment program, went to AA, attended another treatment program, and is now attending AA again.

During all of this, she tells us about her failed relationships, DUIs, and loss of her nursing license. If you have little experience with addicts, you can't help but have a feeling of either pity or scorn for this woman and a sense that treatment for substance use disorders must be quite ineffective.

Melinda's story is not unusual in the number of relapses she has had. Based on her story, it appears that she first had treatment somewhere in the early 1990s. Today, she has 2½ years of sobriety, as far as we know. So, for over 15 to 20 years, she has struggled to manage her disorder. If you believe that addiction is a chronic condition (and I do believe this), it is not surprising to see patients relapse. When you read Melinda's story, it is a hodgepodge of treatment, psychiatric medications, AA, retreats, alternative lifestyle management, school, and relationships. Like many disease concept addicts, she desperately tries to find a way to live a sober lifestyle.

We don't know if Melinda suffers from a co-occurring mental disorder that would have an impact on her recovery. She tells us that a psychiatrist diagnosed her with bipolar disorder and had her on medication. However, she discontinued the medication on her own. She doesn't describe many symptoms of bipolar disorder. She does describe being quite depressed after a period of five years of sobriety, so a depressive disorder cannot be ruled out. The existence of an undiagnosed co-occurring mental disorder would be an explanation as to why she could not achieve continuing sobriety.

CONCLUSION

When you compare Steve's and Melinda's stories, the obvious question is why could Steve achieve long-term sobriety without any slips or relapses through attending AA and why did Melinda need repeated treatment episodes and other interventions after many relapses? After all, they both had significant problems as a result of their alcohol dependence. Is Steve stronger willed or smarter? Does Melinda have co-occurring mental disorders or some other problem that Steve does not?

With regard to a strong will or intelligence, there is no research evidence or my own clinical and personal experience that would support this. In regard to the cases of Steve and Melinda, they both have advanced education and so there is nothing to suggest that one is brighter than the other. In treatment facilities and in Twelve Step support groups, you find people from every socio-economic, ethnic, racial, and professional group. You hear stories like Steve's and stories like Melinda's. Relapse or lack of relapse does not seem connected to any particular demographic character-istic. With regard to strength of will, you would expect that, if Steve was strong willed (in comparison to Melinda), he would have quit drinking long before he did. The reality is that there are disease model addicts who have accomplished a lot, achieved success, and overcome barriers in other areas of their life. You also find disease model addicts who have not. Regardless, it is impossible to establish a relationship to "strength of will" in other areas and relapse occurrences.

The issue of co-occurring mental disorders may be more relevant. As we discussed in Chapter 1, we know that a significant percentage of those who have a substance abuse disorder have a co-occurring mental disorder. For the moment, let's leave out those with antisocial personality disorder, since that will be the focus of an entire chapter of the book. However, it is logical that untreated depressive disorders or anxiety disorders (e.g., post-traumatic stress disorder) or even conditions such as attention-deficit dis-order or a reading disability could be a cause of relapse. Many disease model addicts have masked the symptoms or emotional consequences of a co-occurring disorder through their alcohol and other drug use. Once they discontinue using, there is no way to hide from the symptoms and emotions, and this can lead many disease model addicts to relapse.

Although we don't know if the presence or absence of co-occurring dis-orders can help explain Steve's lack of relapsing and Melinda's frequent relapses, the suspicion that this is a factor is a great example of why sub-stance use disorders require the continuing management and care of pro-fessionals. As Steve's case showed, there are many disease model addicts who maintain continuing sobriety by attending Twelve Step sup-port groups (AA or NA). I hope Melinda finds long-term sobriety in this way too. However, there are many disease model addicts who need addi-tional care and management, especially if there is a co-occurring mental disorder. There are also numerous other issues that can lead to relapse, including financial problems, relationship issues, educational and voca-tional problems, social isolation, and social skill deficits. This means that many or most disease concept addicts need to be in continuing contact with a professional who works with patients with substance use disorders.

If Melinda was a hypertensive woman, she would (hopefully) have regular visits with her healthcare provider, who would monitor her diet, exercise program, stress, and medications. Today, we know that most dis-ease model addicts need the same type of continuing care to manage their condition. If we conceptualize disease model addicts as having a chronic condition that needs the same level of attention as chronic medical condi-tions, relapses might be reduced.

Disease model addicts may be the smallest subtype, but they make up the largest segment of the treatment population. They are probably over-represented in Twelve Step support groups and have demonstrated that, with proper care, they can achieve long-term sobriety. As we will see in the next chapter, the treatment of disease model addicts may be adversely impacted by the inclusion of another subtype of addict: the antisocial personality disorder addict.

THREE

Antisocial Personality Disorder (ASPD)

INTRODUCTION TO AND DEFINITION OF ANTISOCIAL PERSONALITY DISORDER

From reading Chapter 1, you may recall the prominent role of ASPD in two of the subtypes (i.e., Young Antisocial and Chronic Severe). Although there are many different mental disorders that frequently co-occur with substance use disorders (e.g., depressive disorders, anxiety disorders), ASPD is the only personality disorder that is mentioned frequently. According to the *Diagnostic and Statistical Manual of Mental Disorders, Fourth Edition, Text Revision* (DSM-IV TR), "A Personality Disorder is an enduring pattern of inner experience and behavior that deviates markedly from the expectations of the individual's culture, is pervasive and inflexible, has an onset in adolescence or early adulthood, is stable over time, and leads to distress or impairment."[1] The words "enduring pattern," "pervasive and inflexible," and "stable over time" in this definition are indicative of the difficulty in treating personality disorders. These disorders are usually managed rather than treated. With other types of mental disorders, medications are frequently part of the treatment, but that is not the case with personality disorders.

The following criteria from the DSM-IV TR are used to diagnose ASPD:

A. There is a pervasive pattern of disregard for and violation of the rights of others occurring since age 15 years, as indicated by three (or more) of the following:
   (1) failure to conform to social norms with respect to lawful behaviors as indicated by repeatedly performing acts that are grounds for arrest
   (2) deceitfulness as indicated by repeated lying, use of aliases, or conning others for personal profit or pleasure
   (3) impulsivity or failure to plan ahead
   (4) irritability and aggressiveness, as indicated by repeated physical fights or assaults
   (5) reckless disregard for safety of self or others
   (6) consistent irresponsibility, as indicated by repeated failure to sustain consistent work behavior or honor financial obligations
   (7) lack of remorse, as indicated by being indifferent to or rationalizing having hurt, mistreated, or stolen from another
B. The individual is at least 18 years.
C. There is evidence of Conduct Disorder with onset behavior before age 15 years.
D. The occurrence of antisocial behavior is not exclusively during the course of Schizophrenia or Manic Episode.[2]*

For the purposes of this discussion, the important parts of the criteria for ASPD diagnosis are the seven parts of "A." "B" indicates that the individual must be an adult and "C" indicates that there must be evidence by age 15 of behaviors similar to those demonstrated by people with ASPD (The behavioral criteria for conduct disorder are similar to those of ASPD. However, many children and adolescents exhibit these behaviors for other reasons besides ASPD [e.g., emotional trauma, physical or sexual abuse]). With regard to "D," ASPD is not diagnosed if the problem behaviors are due to one of these other disorders.

When you read the descriptions of the seven criteria in "A," it probably occurs to you that you would not want to encounter, let alone have a relationship with, someone who could be diagnosed with ASPD. The terms "psychopath" and "sociopath" have been used in the past to describe people

---

*Reprinted with permission from the *Diagnostic and Statistical Manual of Mental Disorders, Text Revision, Fourth Edition* (Copyright 2000). American Psychiatric Association.

with ASPD. Here is a telling line from the DSM-IV TR when describing the diagnostic process for ASPD: "Because deceit and manipulation are central features of Antisocial Personality Disorder, it may be especially helpful to integrate information acquired from systematic clinical assessment with information collected from collateral sources."[3] In other words, people with ASPD usually lie, so a clinician had better get information from other people to corroborate anything the patient says. According to the DSM-IV TR, ASPD occurs in 3% of males and 1% of females.

TREATMENT OF ASPD

As was stated earlier, personality disorders are difficult to treat, and ASPD is no exception. According to experts in the field, "... while *antisocial* patients are less likely to commit crimes in later life, they continue to be poor spouses, inadequate parents, and unsteady workers. A quarter of them will die prematurely. These findings support the caution of most clinicians about treating these patients [emphasis in original]."[4] "No medications are routinely used or specifically approved for ASP (antisocial personality disorder) treatment. Several drugs, however, have been shown to reduce aggression—a common problem for many antisocials . . . Incarceration may be the best way to control the most severe and persistent cases of antisocial personality disorder."[5] "Antisocial personality disorder is considered one of the most difficult of all personality disorders to treat. Individuals rarely seek treatment on their own and may only initiate therapy when mandated by a court. The efficacy of treatment for antisocial personality disorder is largely unknown."[6]

RELATIONSHIP OF ASPD TO SUBSTANCE USE DISORDERS

Although people with ASPD sound pretty bad and treating such individuals seems dismal, the frequency of this disorder in the general population is quite low. However, if we look at the population of people with a substance use disorder, the prevalence of ASPD is dramatically different. According to a publication by the Center for Substance Abuse Treatment on co-occurring mental disorders, more than 39% of patients in substance abuse treatment had a diagnosis of ASPD. Remember, the prevalence of ASPD in the general population is only 3% for males and 1% for females. Amazingly, nearly 60% of patients who used a combination of alcohol, cocaine, and heroin were diagnosed with ASPD. Compare these percentages of patients with co-occurring ASPD and a substance use disorder to those with other common co-occurring mental disorder such as major depression (12%) or a generalized anxiety disorder (4%) and it is clear that ASPD is a pervasive co-occurring mental disorder among patients in substance abuse treatment.[7]

This information regarding the prevalence of ASPD among patients being treated for a substance use disorder is disturbing for several reasons. First, people with ASPD sound like they are very dangerous and scary individuals when you read the criteria for diagnosing this disorder. Second, the prognosis isn't very positive. Third, the disease model of addiction conceptualizes addiction as an illness and assumes that addicts are just like everyone else, with the exception of having the condition of addiction. If nearly 4 out 10 addicts have ASPD, this sizeable minority of addicts certainly aren't just like everyone else.

Since the implications of having so many addicts with ASPD are significant, it is useful to examine the prevalence data more closely. According to too many "prevalence" the DSM-IV TR, the prevalence of ASPD is very low in the general population, but it is three times higher among males than among females. According to the 2007 report of admissions to treatment (latest report available), nearly 68% of admissions were male and 32% were female.[8] So, there would be some expectation that the prevalence of ASPD among the treatment population would be higher than in the general population, but it still should not exceed the 3% prevalence among males. A better explanation may be found in the source of referral to treatment. In 2007, 37.5% of referrals to treatment came from the criminal justice system.[9] When you examine the criteria to diagnose ASPD, it is clear that people with ASPD are very likely to come into contact with the criminal justice system. Now, some of these referrals from the criminal justice system are for driving under the influence (DUI), and it could be argued that people arrested for DUI are no more likely to have ASPD than anyone else. However, previous reports of treatment admissions indicate that only about 7.5% of these criminal justice referrals are for DUI.[10] In addition, we have to consider age, since ASPD cannot be diagnosed before the age of 18. In 2006, 11.7% of the treatment admissions were in the age range of 12 to 19 years, and over half of the admissions of adolescents (age 12 to 17) were from the criminal justice system.[11, 12] Therefore, although we can't be completely precise due to the age overlap, less than 6% of the total criminal justice referrals to treatment probably came from an age group too young to be diagnosed with ASPD. If we combine this with the percentage of criminal justice referrals for DUI, we have accounted for about a third of the referrals from the criminal justice system (i.e., of the 37.5% of the referrals from the criminal justice system, about 6% are adolescents and about 7.5% were for DUI.

That is 13.5% or about a third of the total of the referrals from the criminal justice system). However, that still means, even with this conservative estimate, that about a quarter of all the referrals to treatment (i.e., 37.5% minus 13.5%, or 24%) came from criminal justice systems, which probably have a lot of "clients" with ASPD. This would certainly be a major explanation for the reason why so many patients in substance abuse treatment have ASPD.

Finally, a reason why there are so many patients with ASPD in treatment probably has to do with the fact that people with ASPD are very likely to use and abuse alcohol and other drugs. According to an epidemiological survey by the National Institute of Mental Health, 83.6% of individuals with ASPD demonstrated some form of substance abuse.[13]

It is quite easy to see the relationship between the criteria for a substance abuse disorder and the criteria for ASPD. Recall from Chapter 1 that the criteria for a substance abuse disorder include "failure to fulfill major role obligations," and one of the ASPD criteria is "consistent irresponsibility." Physical fights are mentioned as indications of irritability and aggressiveness for ASPD and as an example of "persistent or recurrent social or interpersonal problems" for a substance abuse disorder. The fifth criterion for ASPD is "reckless disregard for the safety of self or others" and the second criterion for a substance abuse disorder is using substances in situations that are physically hazardous. Legal problems are mentioned in the criteria for both conditions.

Since there is a great deal of similarity between the criteria for ASPD and a substance abuse disorder, it is reasonable to wonder if many substance abusers are misdiagnosed as ASPD. Theoretically, that should not happen because a careful assessment would gather information throughout the client's childhood and adolescent history and that would distinguish those with ASPD and a substance use disorder from those with a substance use disorder but without ASPD. However, in the real world, assessments may not be that careful or thorough and, therefore, there may be some danger of over-diagnosing ASPD among substance use disorder treatment populations. If you have ever worked in a substance abuse treatment or recovery setting, you know that the things many addicts without ASPD do during the time they are using alcohol and other drugs are very similar to the things that people with ASPD do. Once there is a period of sobriety, it is often easier to discriminate between those patients in treatment who have ASPD from those who do not. The patients without ASPD are often filled with guilt and remorse over the things they have done to others, while those with ASPD are indifferent to their actions or just seem to be intellectually aware of them but emotionally detached from them. Therefore, treatment providers often can only determine which patients really have ASPD after a period of sobriety.

IMPLICATIONS FOR SUBSTANCE ABUSE TREATMENT

As we saw in Chapter 1, less than half of those who enter treatment actually complete it. However, let's examine the treatment-completion data more closely. First, we are going to exclude all of those who only go through detoxification. Detoxification is just a period of time that the patient is in a controlled environment and not using alcohol or other drugs. It is often referred to as "drying out." After detoxification, the patient might be transferred to treatment, but detoxification itself is not really treatment. So, excluding patients in detoxification, about 55% of patients in treatment either completed it or were transferred to some other type of treatment than the one they entered initially.[14] Treatment is classified according to the level of service and can be outpatient, intensive outpatient, short-term residential, long-term residential, hospital-residential, or outpatient medically assisted opioid therapy (e.g., methadone). Outpatient and intensive outpatient treatment are conducted in free-standing treatment facilities where the patient just spends part of a day or evening and are differentiated from each other by how many hours a day and days a week the patient spends in treatment. Obviously, intensive outpatient involves more hours a day and/or more days per week than outpatient. Outpatient treatment is by far the most frequent type of service provided. One reason for that is that it is the cheapest type of service. Short-term residential, long-term residential, and hospital-residential are provided in settings where the patient spends 24 hours a day.

Now, it would be expected that patients referred to treatment from the criminal justice system would have high treatment completion or transfer rates. After all, these patients are ordered to treatment by the criminal justice system and, if they fail in treatment, there is usually some kind of adverse consequence (i.e., incarceration) that will be imposed. While patients referred by the criminal justice system do complete treatment at a higher rate than those referred by other sources, it still isn't very high. For example, only 58% of criminal justice referred patients completed (or transferred from) outpatient treatment.[15] That is higher than the 42.8% completion for self-referrals or the 46% completion for referrals from the community,[16] but it still doesn't seem very high for patients under sanctions from the criminal justice system.

Of course, we don't know how many of the patients referred from the criminal justice system have ASPD. Two studies showed very similar prevalence rates for ASPD of around 47% for criminal justice popula-tions.[17, 18] So, we can assume that nearly half of these patients referred by the criminal justice system have ASPD. This would certainly explain why so many of these patients fail to complete treatment even though they have sanctions from the criminal justice system. Remember that the crite-ria for diagnosing ASPD include impulsivity, irresponsibility, and lack of remorse. These characteristics are not the ones you would associate with completing substance abuse treatment.

This is not meant to say that ASPD is the only reason for patients to fail to complete treatment. The rate of treatment completion for those who are referred from other sources is even lower than for those referred from the criminal justice system. Of course, some proportion of these referrals could also have ASPD, but patients frequently terminate treatment simply because it is very difficult for them to abstain from alcohol and other drugs. We know that people with chronic conditions that must be managed through lifestyle changes (e.g., hypertension, diabetes) have very low rates of treatment compliance. The same is true for patients with substance use disorders. It is very difficult to make the lifestyle changes needed to maintain an alcohol and other drug-free life. Or, the patients may have other co-occurring mental disorders that, if not treated, are barriers to treatment.

There is at least circumstantial evidence that ASPD could be a significant factor in the high rates of treatment failure for patients in substance abuse treatment. However, there is also the disruption that ASPD can have on the treatment process for everyone. Let's just imagine that you are a drug and alcohol counselor working in a public-sector outpatient treatment program for men (i.e., a program that receives state and federal funds to operate and serves those without the ability to pay). You don't have a lot of formal counselor training but you've been in recovery for a long time so you know what your patients have been through. Now, this kind of work is tough under any circumstances. People get to your program through different sources but no one is happy to be there. The patients have suffered a lot of consequences as a result of their alcohol and other drug use, so many of them realize that they need help. But, this may be the first time in years that many of them have been abstinent for more than a day or two. Initially, they may be feeling physically uncomfortable as their bodies adjust to not having alcohol and other drugs. They have a lot of problems involving personal relationships, money, and the law. So, for the first week to 10 days, everyone feels bad. You run a group for 10 guys. After about a week, about half the guys start coming to grips with their problems and demonstrate a desire to do the work necessary to get better. But, the other half of the guys are disruptive. They don't seem to take responsibility for their problems, they come late to group, and they make disparaging comments about you and the other people in the group. Some of them are hostile and menacing.

It is likely that many or most of the disruptive group members have ASPD. But, how can the counselor help the other group members when half the group acts like that? So, the disruptive patients will probably get kicked out eventually but, meanwhile, they are adversely impacting the treatment of those who are motivated to get better.

The point here is that many of the problems in substance abuse treatment, especially in public-sector treatment, may be due to the large numbers of patients with ASPD. In the final chapter of the book, we will discuss ways of handling the ASPD patient.

CASE EXAMPLES

Henry's Story

I was born the son of two well-educated, fairly affluent parents. Neither one drank or had any connection with drug use. I had one older sister and one older brother. My sister graduated from a private girl's school, is married to a professional engineer and has one child. My brother graduated from a military academy, the same as my father. He has two children and he and his family live a fulfilling life. My father was a funeral director, a business established in 1873 and passed down through family generations. By most accounts, my father was a likeable guy and was quite successful. He was a full colonel in the army and commanding officer for our state National Guard. He was a member of the Masons, Rotary Club and countless other organizations. He was also the chairman of the board for the state funeral directors. Although the business was passed down for many generations, my father did not encourage any of his children to be a part of the business. In fact, he did not want any of us around the funeral home. My brother or sister would have been a good fit in the family business but not me. I was a hell raiser from the start. None of us were close to my father. However, my mom more or less made up for that. She was a stay-at-home mom and attentive to our upbringing. She attended school functions and other activities. While I was considered to have great potential, I was certainly the most problematic for my parents. There was 12 years between my sister and I and four years between my brother and I. While my siblings were very obedient and conforming, I was a constant challenge to my father's authority. The others never got in trouble but I was constantly at odds with my dad and his rules. I have no doubt that I was a disappointment. I remember when I was 15 I took money I had saved up from summer jobs and bought a Honda motorcycle. When my father found out, he took the bike and sold it. I never saw the bike or money again. Of course, it should be noted that I was forbidden to buy or ride a motorcycle. I only got away with it for two weeks. He found where the bike was hidden and the rest is history. At the age of 16, shortly after I got my license, I was involved in an accident. I lost control of the vehicle I was driving. I hit one of my school friend's little sister. She died at the scene. From that moment on, my friend and his family's life changed forever as well as my own life and my family. My attorney at the time proved that the tie rod had snapped which was consistent with my claim that I lost steering as I entered the curve where the accident occurred. The prosecutor claimed the tie rod had snapped as a result of the accident when the car came to rest in a culvert. In the end, I was found guilty of involuntary manslaughter and sentenced to 11 to 23 months in county jail. Since I was under 18, I was housed in a segregated cell and left to myself. In time, I was allowed out to mop floors and then eventually I was allowed to attend school after which I had to go straight back to my cell. The father of the little girl I hit had a terrible time trying to cope with the loss of child. As you can well imagine, he was never quite the same. One day, as I was walking from school to jail, he found me and ran his car up on the sidewalk and almost got me. About two weeks later, I was cutting the grass at the back of the jail. I had stopped the mower to fill it with gas. I heard someone yelling at me, "You are a murderer." I turned to look and there was the dad standing at the edge of the yard. I was seventeen at that time and not afraid of much. But I surely thought I was going to be shot that day. I knelt down to the mower and tried to pretend I didn't hear him and go about my work. But, he was not going to be put off. He continued to yell at me. All I could do was tell him it was an accident and that I didn't want it to happen any more than he did. With that, he charged me. I got him off of me but he simply got back up and started hitting me again. I didn't want to fight this guy. If I were him, I might well have done the same thing. I tried to make my way back to the jail's back door knowing that I would have to ring the bell to get back in. Just as I got to the door, it opened. Out came the warden and a guard and they grabbed the dad and took me back inside. I was sure that the story would get turned around and somehow it would all be made out to be my fault. But as it turned out, the warden had been watching me from his office window and saw and heard the entire incident. About two weeks later, they decided to remand me to the custody of my parents and a form of probation. I found out later that they had decided they did not want to be responsible for my safety and so decided to let my parents deal with it. At any rate, there were lines that were drawn in our little community between those who saw it one way and those who viewed it another. I finished high school and headed for college. My second year of college, my mom fell ill with some unknown ailment. She woke up one morning and no longer had use of her hands or legs. They tried everything but she passed away a short time later. Eleven months after that, my dad dropped over dead and that was that. I didn't know it at the time, but I was completely lost. The house was sold, the business was sold and what seemed like any connection to family or security I had known was gone. There were too many sad memories in that little town. So I moved on to [name of city]. No particular reason, other than I had a friend who lived there and I wanted to head to [name of part of the country] and see the world. Once in [name of city], I worked a couple odd jobs and then invested what money I had from my inheritance into a club. The nightclub was a major headache and didn't pull in the money I had hoped for. I sold it and opened a tanning salon and carwash. Everything was okay except for my choices. Growing up in the sixties, I had experimented with all kinds of drugs. I was never one for the heavy stuff like heroin or needles. I didn't like coke but I smoked my share of weed and did the LSD thing. What I really liked was speed. I had done my share of it when I was a teenager and in my twenties. But I had more or less left it behind by the time I had gone to [name of city]. The thing was, I knew how to make it. That was the cash flow opportunity of a lifetime in [name of city] and I simply didn't have the sense to pass it up. I started out small and was such a success that I had everyone asking where that stuff came from. Eventually I was asked to meet this guy. A friend of a friend kind of thing. Apparently my work had caught the eye of some big players and before you knew it, I was flying to [name of state]. I was set up there with a state of the art lab. Make a hundred pounds, get $100,000. Meanwhile fly first class, enjoy the [name of place] and live like a king. It all seemed great at first. By the time the product reached the streets, it had been diluted 70 percent and we still couldn't keep up with demand. The problem of course was I enjoyed my own product and it was as pure as the driven snow. Clearly, I didn't make the best choices when I was without the addition of a strong pharmaceutical in my system. At this point, I would be up for three or four days at a time without sleep. I was running back and forth from [name of city] to [name of city]. Thinking I could do it all. All I was doing was kidding myself while going deep into an addiction. I was digging a hole that would take years to crawl out of. It wasn't long before the house of cards came tumbling down. Someone got arrested and, contrary to the myth, there is no honor among thieves. The idea of keeping your mouth shut went away with the original boys in the mafia. Let's face it, even they gave each other up in the end. The DEA and authorities in general want the guy at the top or at least as close as they can get. Ultimately, that quest led to me. By this time, I had been getting away with this activity for years. Needless to say, I had amassed quite a collection of assets. Two homes, seven expensive collector automobiles, a plane, a thirty foot cigarette boat, a motorcycle and on and on. I collected guns, watches and fine time pieces. I even had a mini casino in my game room, complete with table games and slots. It was all rather outrageous. Technically, I had all my ducks in a row. I had two legitimate businesses with exaggerated incomes. I made sure the IRS got theirs. I wasn't dealing drugs. The place I made the stuff was thousands of miles away from my home. There was nothing to connect me, except of course the addiction. Having an addiction, means there must be a source. It is paramount that nothing interferes with your supply. Over the years, I had compiled quite an abundance of methamphetamine. I had always planned to stop manufacturing one day. So of course, I needed to make sure that I would have all I needed to see me into the foreseeable future. Hence, therein lies the rub. The DEA is quite methodical in their efforts to turn every stone, so to speak. While they had no luck searching my home or businesses, they did uncover the fact that I had a storage locker. I thought I had that one covered too. The storage locker had chemicals stored in it for the carwash business. Nothing they could find there! I thought I had been quite clever with regards to the concealment of my "stash." In order to get to that, you had to remove the back wall of the storage unit which would put you into another unit all together. That one wasn't in my name. The proper entrance to that unit was on the other side of the building. Besides, I would think you would need a whole different search warrant to go into someone else's storage unit! THE BEST LAID PLANS, OF MICE AND ADDICTS. Even the affable federal agent was impressed with that one! What he wasn't impressed by was the all so predictable behavior of just another drug user. Tired of having to remove every single screw each and every time I needed access to my stash, I left a few screws loose. The drill gun on the floor didn't help much either. At any rate, there is this pesky thing called "reasonable cause." My fate was sealed. There were lawyers and fees and negotiations. They were certain that I had obtained the drugs from a major supplier they had recently dismantled. That idea worked for me. I couldn't offer any more than myself anyway. Giving up the people I was involved with would have earned me a fate worse than a prison sentence. So I took the lumps. Ten to life, commuted to a flat ten years. With programs and good time I could whittle that down to just over five. Once inside I became a law clerk. I worked on a double jeopardy angle to get me out. Everything I owned was seized. Plus I was in prison. It seemed like I had been punished twice for the same crime. Turns out, the DEA seized my property but the state was the arresting agency. The Supreme Court handed down a decision saying that since the United States and my state of residency are two different sovereigns, each only punished me once even though there were two punishments for the same crime. The punishments were a single act by two different sovereigns. Therefore, double jeopardy did not exist. STRIKE TWO! I still had one more shot. The DEA only took the really valuable stuff like the houses and the cars. The state still had all my furnishings and other items in impound. Since the state had property of mine that they had also seized that was clearly double jeopardy by the same sovereign. I had them! By decree of the highest court in our land, I was on solid ground. I challenged the state in court. Rather than release me, they elected to release the property. By this time, years had gone by. Looking for a bright spot amid all this gloom, I told myself that at least I could sell my belongings and have money to start out with when I got out. So I made arrangements to have a friend secure two moving trucks and go pick my stuff up at [the] police impound. The day he arrived, there wasn't anything to pick up. The police said my attorney came and got the stuff for me. What attorney? I fired my attorney five years ago! SOME CROOKS WEAR A SUIT AND TIE! Seems my ex attorney had found himself in debt. The gentlemen he owed operated out of [name of city]. I filed all the necessary paperwork and settled down to wait for the slow wheels of justice to turn. Then, as I sat in my cell one morning the guard came to get me and said, "The FBI are here and want to talk to you." WOW! The FBI. This guy is really in trouble now! So down I went to a little room in the prison. There were two agents inside. I had a seat. I inquired, "How can I help you?" The reply was, you can start by telling us who you had shoot your attorney. Apparently, after spending several hours at a favorite strip club in [name of city], he was shot in route to his car. "He is in critical condition and not expected to live," I was told. "We know what he did; your little 'situation' regarding the theft of your property. That was the straw that broke the camel's back, wasn't it? You were not going to stand for that, huh? So you reached out and had it taken care of, didn't you?" All I could think, was, uh oh! This isn't good, this isn't good at all. Round and round we went. Good cop, bad cop. Question after question. The thing about the truth is, it doesn't change. Finally, they left vowing to be back. Two days later, they found the guy who shot him and it was all due to a gambling debt. HE LIVED! I pursued my case against him, even as he recovered. He was stripped of his bar license and ordered to pay me $182,000. He would not be permitted to practice law again until he had made restitution. I never saw the money and he doesn't practice law. He sells wheel chairs for a living now. The only thing I had left was the fact that I was getting out soon and the state bar of [name of state] was sending me $5,000 from their client's security fund because of my dealings with such an unscrupulous lawyer practicing in their state. True to their word, two weeks before I got out, a check for five thousand dollars was put on my books at prison. At least, I had some money to start a new life with. The day I got out, the prison cut me a check for $241. What! Where's the $5,000 the state bar sent me? I was told, this is it, less my room and board over the years that the prison was keeping. STRIKE THREE, YOU'RE OUT! And so I was. Out, that is. I went to 47 job interviews before I got hired to deliver office goods. I wasn't in prison but a few months before I made the decision to never do drugs again. It's been 15 years of clean and sober for me. Never once stepped back or relapsed. But that's not to say that drugs haven't affected my life since. One of the jobs I have had in the years since was being the director of a sober living home helping those whose lives had been impacted by drug and alcohol use. Part of being an addict in recovery is to remain vigilant regarding your addictive nature. Many addicts tend to replace one addiction with another. I was aware of this so I thought to myself that if I kept really busy, I wouldn't have time to slip back into my problem. I focused on working. It wasn't long before someone referred to me as a workaholic. I found it a bit ironic that I was still serving an addiction. At least this obsession would not have any legal ramifications. However, in my quest to do the right thing I met a girl, who somehow or someway reached deep inside me and gained my undivided attention. Struggling with familiar issues, I felt qualified and compelled to help her. I lost sight of the fact that you can only help those who want to help themselves. We got married. Her commitment to sobriety was fleeting. She would do well for awhile and then relapse. I found myself where most family members of addicts tend to find themselves. Although I had been clean and sober for years at this point, my whole life was being swept up dealing with addiction. Only this time, I was going to truly experience the effects that the addict has on their loved ones: the broken promises, the hope and the betrayal. There were countless hours of worrying and frustration. I got her into therapy several times. I set her up with drug counselors and meetings. But the story was always the same in the end. Finally, in a last effort, I quit my job and sold my home and we moved to [name of state] where

I went to work in management for the [name of company]. I also took a job at a sober-living home, called [name of recovery house]. Both were basically full time jobs. I lived on the property at the [name of sober living house] and would commute from there to my job with [name of company]. Of course it was my hope that having my wife in close proximity to a treatment program would have its benefits. Again, I was diligent in my efforts to guide her through recovery. I helped her get a job and placed her on the path. Life is such that we all have our share of tragedies. Addicts will always be quick to point out theirs. These tragedies are generally the preferred excuses when explaining yet another relapse. In my wife's case, her former marriage was to an individual from [name of country]. When they were married, they actually lived in [name of country] for a period of time. At one point, when they were back here in the U.S.A., the husband took their two children and fled back to [name of country]. The youngest child was only months old. Since the children were born in [name of country], try as she might, she had no hope of getting the children back. It would be years before she saw her children again. By then, she had fallen into a state of depression which ultimately led her to drug use. By the time she was reunited with her children, they were teenagers. They had been raised in [name of country]. Based on what they had been taught, there was little respect for women from her offsprings. Their mother had abandoned them and was a worthless human being. When her opportunity came to finally see her children again, the kids were so jaded that her dreams were once again dashed. And so, this was another excellent opportunity to slip deeper into addiction. Unlike all the other addicts I had worked with, I was deeply involved in her life. Try as I might, I was unable to remain detached enough to make the hard decisions that I normally would with others. I kept on trying to "fix her" until I simply admitted to myself that I just couldn't do it. I could go no further. I was completely and utterly worn out. And so, it ended. She was gone and back to the people, places and things where she felt comfortable. She really ended up with nowhere to go. She stayed with friends, slept in her car and kept right on feeding her addiction. Finally, she met a fellow who took her in. The story that was relayed to me was that he was wealthy and she was doing well. The reality of it was that he was deeply involved in drug transporting in and out of [name of country]. The details are vague. However, the end result for her was an arrest and incarceration. At the time I am writing this, she has been in prison for a year and a half and still waiting to be sentenced. I was unable to save her. Maybe this will. It is my hope, that she has reached her "rock bottom" and perhaps, will be able to start a better way of life once she gets out. Only time, will tell. As for me, I have had the education of seeing more than just the side of the actual addict. It is honestly hard to recall all that went on while you were deep in your addiction, anyway. Despite your deepest soul searching, you just can't or don't want to remember it all. There were a number of times that my wife, by her actions, was able to jog my memory with regard to things I had done but forgotten. In the long run, it all served to strengthen my own recovery. I believe that the challenges I had to face with my wife were more than most recovering addicts could take. Yet, through it all, I remained clean and sober. However, the fact remains that my life was once again severely affected by drugs and addiction, even if it wasn't my own use of drugs. As for my "choices," that clearly is still a work in progress.

I live a pretty simple life now. I have a small business and I make my way. I would attribute my success to getting back to common sense and most of all the help of one individual who ran a program in the prison I was located at. A no nonsense, tough old bird who really pissed me off until I grew to love him like a father. Always told it like it is, even though a lot of it was stuff I didn't want to hear. He made me face my fears and honor my commitments. I live by his example to this day. He showed me the way and then kicked my ass down the road a few times. To make sure I kept moving ahead, he gave me a saying to live by: "Everything I need is already in me." Thanks [name of person]. You're the best. I have been blessed as well by the fact that I do not struggle with my addiction on a day- to-day basis. That is to say, I do not long for the drug as once I did. It all seems pretty far behind me now. My life in the fast lane was something else. There was a lot to be attracted to. For me it was the lifestyle, the money and the high. I was living like a rock star. But when I look back at my fall from grace, it was a long time going down. While the good times seemed to rush right by, the consequences dragged on for an eternity. It had a profound effect on my health, those that I loved and my own quality of life as a whole. When I think of revisiting that rush of doing meth, I immediately replace it with the memories of living in the abyss; where it got me and what I gave away as a consequence. I think of long nights living in a cell and knocking roaches off my bed as I tried to sleep. I think of the countless individuals whom I have worked with whose lives and loved ones were impacted far worse than mine. Some of us never make it back. In my case, I was part of a program in prison that had just got off the ground. This particular program was called [name of program]. Unlike most do-it-yourself, half-hearted attempts put in place by most institutions, this program was a 24/7 life experience in recovery. The selected inmates were housed in a separate building. There were approximately 100 of us. We lived together and we ate together. Right after breakfast, we would have a meeting. The rest of the day was then filled with classes such as critical thinking, parenting and many classes on drugs, alcohol and their affects. Moreover, there was a group meeting every day. We were all split into smaller groups. These groups were much more intimate with approximately a dozen or so individuals. What was discussed in these groups was completely private. If you were caught talking out of school so to speak, you were ejected from the program. It was in these groups that I believe the most progress was made. Each group became very tight. A common bond was established among these men. We knew each other's secrets; what had brought them to their current place in life. Eventually, you were able to break through even the toughest of the hard cases. Everyone in the group would take a vested interest in helping a fellow group member. When something would happen on the outside that would have an effect on any one group member's mental and emotional state, we would all be aware of it. The effected individual would not be allowed to wallow in his anguish. Everyone would chip in to see to it. Whoever needed attention got it. This was basically the same principle as NA or AA. However, there was no leaving the meeting and going home. Your interaction with fellow [name of program] members was intense. Each evening after dinner your day would end with a NA/AA meeting. We even had speakers come in from the outside. The program was six months long. As I mentioned earlier, I was in prison about six months when I realized I could never do drugs again. The [name of the program] program was at the end of my sentence. One might think that since I already hit rock bottom and I knew I simply could not be involved in drugs again perhaps I didn't need the program. I can tell you that would be inaccurate. Knowing what you need to do is a good first step. But, you still need the tools to build a new life. You need the knowledge to build the bridge. That is where [name of the program] and/or NA/AA comes in. It is your technical school complete with all the tools you will need. The only ingredient missing is your commitment. That one is completely on you! If you attend AA or NA meetings without commitment, in the long run, you're only fooling yourself. There is an old A.A. saying that goes "Fake it till you make it!" that may be helpful in the beginning. But, the emphasis needs to remain on the make it, not fake it. In the end, it really comes down to how sick and tired you are of being sick and tired. How committed you really are. How sincere you are with regard to the damage you have done to those who love you and have tried to help you. All that being said, above all, you have to do it for yourself. Being an addict means you have become an expert at letting yourself down. You have mastered the ability to take the easy way out, none of which is going to look that impressive in your resume for life or character. Recovery isn't easy. For most addicts, it is the toughest thing they will ever attempt. It's a day to day struggle for the rest of your life for most. The payoff is that you'll actually have a life. It may even save your life or someone else's. There certainly is no shortage of deaths caused by drunk drivers. There is no doubt that the program I was involved in was the supporting factor for my success to this point. Many of the things I learned and experienced in that program help me to this day. It prepared me for what I would face once I got out of prison. Without it, I don't know that I would have been properly prepared to deal with the adjustments that were needed once I was released. It is my understanding that due to fiscal shortages, that program is no longer offered. It honestly worries me regarding what will happen to all the inmates that will not have the advantage of that kind of program. Certainly, they will need to build more prison space. For I am sure, without that kind of help, most of them will be back. It is my position that state and federal agencies need to look at what works and what doesn't. The recidivism rate for graduates of programs like the one I was involved in are substantially lower. It is simply a matter of common sense, as I see it. You can spend the money on programs. Or you can build more prisons. The programs are going to change lives for the better; save lives and make productive citizens out of drug offenders. I am living proof of that. The alternative they are going to learn is how to survive and live in prison. Believe me, they will bring those skills back to the street. Especially the younger ones. They are easily influenced if there is no alternative source of education. We are simply breeding a cancer that will eventually consume this country from the inside out. A few weeks before I was set to graduate from [name of program], I was asked to write something that I would read to the graduating class. The following is what I read on the day of graduation. It sums up my feelings, regarding [name of program] and the importance of programs in prison.

THE ESSENCE OF RECOVERY

The ground that prisons stand on is different in many ways. Etched by paths of fallen men with heavy debts to pay. The days and nights spent on this turf are wrought with aimless time. Hope that springs eternal is an item hard to find. For those who seek the wisdom, their quest will lead to [name of program]. As if amid the desert, guided to the spring. Thus, we have been the fortunate, those who are truly blessed. Tired of living the lives we led, lost and in distress. We came together in search of the cure. Then once accepted, found much to endure. Some did not make it and fell by the way. Those seeking change sit before you today. For the essence of recovery is found within the heart. Like all things that are dear to us, it is here we made our start. Through program and compassion, twelve steps, day by day. We come to graduation having finally found our way. No longer lost, we gather. No longer, fallen men. For with our higher power, we have the strength to stand again and with this new found fortitude, we have the seed to sow. As we are now the influence, our legacy starts to grow. For now our hearts are open. With honor, we strike the bond. Ready for the challenge of recovery and beyond.

While the public in general, may be largely apathetic towards those in prison. I can tell you from first-hand knowledge. You have DUI camps that are full of offenders. A vast majority of inmates are incarcerated on simple drug charges. They were in possession or committed a crime that can be traced back to their addiction. One thing I know for certain; without the programs and the efforts made by those involved, my life would not be as blessed as it is today. That is why I feel it is such a travesty that the particular program I was involved in is no longer available to those inside. While I am sure there are still programs available, they are generally the kind of thing where you simply attend a class once or twice a week or work at a computer and answer questions in a test form. There is a vast difference. The answers to the computer questions are simply traded on the yard. Two or three hours a week in class simply puts you back in the mix of the general population the rest of the time. I am sure that it is no surprise to anyone that there are plenty of drugs in prison. The testing is very random. Like anything else, there is a way around it. A program such as [name of program] was very regimented. Everyone was tested on a regular basis. You were in a recovery program 24/7 much the same as being in a treatment center or an inpatient rehabilitation arrangement. No doubt, there was a substantial expense to operate such a program. However, I would submit the fact that, like any productive citizen, I have spent the past ten years of my life paying income, school, city and all the taxes that help to fund such endeavors. Moreover, as a normal law abiding citizen, I remain out of prison and therefore save the taxpayers $30,000–$40,000 a year for my incarceration. No matter how you get there, be it N.A., A.A., by your own doing or with the help of twelve steps and others, your commitment is the key factor. As over simple as it may sound, once you stop, never, ever, start again. Not under any circumstance. No matter what else may happen in your life. There simply is no good excuse.

Analysis of Henry

First, let's be sure that Henry meets the criteria for ASPD in the DSM-IV TR. Keep in mind that Henry is attempting to create a favorable impression so he is not telling us all the sordid details of his life. However, part of the Twelve Step program of recovery does involve an inventory of past transgressions. So, he does tell us about some of the things he has done. As with most of the case studies, I do have information about the individuals beyond what is contained in their stories or interviews.

If you recall from the description at the beginning of the chapter, to be diagnosed as ASPD, the person must, since the age of 15, demonstrate three or more of the seven attributes. The first one is clear. Henry participated in unlawful behavior repeatedly and eventually was incarcerated. He doesn't say much about the second criterion, which involves deceitfulness. He tells a story about trying to hide his motorcycle from his parents but not much else, apart from the obvious need for a person to lie when he is manufacturing methamphetamine. Although we cannot discern whether Henry meets this criterion from his story, I assure readers that he has a long history of lying and conning people for personal profit. The third criterion involves impulsivity and failure to plan ahead. I would say that these characteristics are not typical for Henry. He demonstrated planning in hiding his supply of methamphetamine and in attempting to launder his drug profits. Similarly, he is not a particularly aggressive individual in regard to getting in fights (fourth criterion). However, Henry certainly meets the fifth criterion. He manufactured methamphetamine, a very dangerous activity, and he was associated with major drug distributors, so he definitely showed a disregard for his safety. The next criterion involves irresponsibility. Although we would expect Henry to show evidence of irresponsibility, he doesn't really tell us much to support this in his story and I don't have any compelling evidence either. Being an illicit drug manufacturer is not exactly demonstrating social responsibility, but it sounds like he produced what he was supposed to produce. The final criterion is the most obvious in Henry's story. His lack of remorse is remarkable and will be discussed more thoroughly later in this section. Therefore, Henry has demonstrated at least four of the seven criteria. The other relevant part of the diagnostic criteria in Henry's case is that there must be some evidence of a conduct disorder before the age of 15. Basically, a conduct disorder means that a person acts like someone with ASPD but is too young to be diagnosed. According to Henry's own story, he caused problems for his family during his childhood. I don't think that there is any question regarding the accuracy of the ASPD diagnosis.

Henry's story is instructive for a couple of reasons. First, it provides a look inside the thinking of someone with ASPD. Second, it shows that a person with ASPD can be convinced to avoid alcohol and other drugs if the consequences are significant enough. With regard to Henry's thinking, let's first focus on the issue of remorse. More than anything, I think this shows the difference between ASPD addicts and any other person, including other addicts. Remember, as he tells this story, he has been sober (according to his account) for many years. He relates a story about how, at the age of 16, he tragically kills his friend's sister in a traffic accident. While Henry tells us that it changed his life, he never says anything about the event being devastating for him. He says that his attorney "proved" that the accident was caused by a mechanical failure in the car but the jury didn't buy it. Now, I don't know about you but if I had been involved in something like this, I would have been racked with guilt for years, regardless of whose fault it was. Henry seems to have avoided this feeling. It is the impact on his life that is of greatest concern to him (i.e., his belief that he was unfairly convicted and had to serve time). While Henry can understand the victim's father's anger at him, he seems emotionally disconnected from it. After he is released to his parents' custody, this life-changing event is never mentioned again. We see this same lack of emotional connection to people when he describes the death of his parents. He describes his parents without any affect ("By most accounts, my father was a likeable guy . . ." and "She was a stay-at-home mom and attentive to our upbringing. She attended school functions and other activities."). Both parents die within a year and he is "completely lost." That is the extent of his description of the trauma of losing both of his parents. Although he has two older siblings, he never mentions them after this initial description. In fact, Henry does not describe any emotional attachment to another person until he tells us about the addict he married. This inability to form emotional attachments or to experience remorse is quite characteristic of ASPD.

The other interesting part of peeking into Henry's world view involves his outrage at the injustices done to him without any regard for his role in creating the situations that led to these perceived injustices. He works diligently to correct the "injustices," and he believes that it is unfair when he doesn't prevail. While incarcerated, he spends a great deal of time on the concept of "double jeopardy" and is appalled when the state takes his assets to pay part of the cost to taxpayers of his incarceration. He is upset that the attorney who ripped him off has not provided restitution. Now, all of Henry's assets were acquired through illegal activity. So, the usual reaction of the public and law enforcement to his "injustices" would be, "So what? You got what you deserved." Henry, however, wants us to appreciate the unfairness of these situations (e.g., "SOME CROOKS WEAR A SUIT AND TIE!"). There is nothing is his story that suggests Henry understands that it was his illegal activity that caused all of these problems.

It may seem counterintuitive that someone like Henry would establish long-term sobriety and stay involved in Twelve Step recovery. I don't want to criticize Henry's recovery program in any way. Regardless of his diagnosis, it is much better to have him sober than not. Whatever his motivation, it is preferable to have him productively employed than committing crimes. Henry tells us that he avoids returning to drug use by thinking about what happened to him. In other words, the threat to his well-being is sufficient to keep him sober. Very concisely, this is what a treatment provider hopes to accomplish with ASPD addicts. In other words, if ASPD addicts meet their needs through alcohol and other drug use, they will experience severe consequences that will prevent them from meeting all of their other needs. This technique does not tend to do so well with ASPD addicts who are impulsive and violent. One reason that ASPD addicts can find satisfaction working in recovery house settings (as Henry did) is that they get to impart their experience, act "tough" with new patients, and get some status in this environment. Whether or not ASPD patients have internalized the message of recovery (i.e., what Henry says at the end of his story about commitment to sobriety), what is important is that they act as if they have internalized it.

Rick's Story

I was born to a single parent in [name of city] which in the 1970s and 80s, especially being in the inner city, was the norm, as was growing up without a black father figure. A lot of the kids I knew didn't have fathers. So, the "street guys" and athletes were who we admired and emulated. My mom was not experienced in raising a child, yet. But, she was an educated black woman; she was a school teacher in [the name of the school district]. She worked hard and gave me all the love and energy that a single mother could give. She was loving, attentive, and generous, yet stern and would deliver a good ass-whooping if she deemed it necessary.

Life for me at a young age was great. I wasn't introduced to any form of drugs until I was 12. Ironically, it was my grandmother, who smoked trees (weed). For as long as I can remember she would puff during the day and before she would go to bed. It was with my grandmother that I smoked weed for my first time, during a football game. For my first time ever I felt the sensation that weed brings, and I liked it. From that day on I smoked as often as I could.

I played all the major sports, football, baseball, and some basketball. I wanted to be an athlete. I would play everything, everyday. I would play anytime, anywhere. That was the one thing about weed; it didn't affect my affinity for sports.

I started drinking about six months after my first taste of weed. My grandmother, uncles, and mom all drank. My grandmother and one of my uncles were alcoholics. My first drink was with my homie, may he Rest In Peace. My first taste was a forty ounce of Old English 800, I didn't really like it, at first. But, as I drank and smoked more I realized I liked it. I was becoming addicted. I started off drinking a forty ounce now and then. Like my sports when I was a kid, it became an anytime, anywhere activity. I was drinking and smoking everyday. "High" and "tipsy" was my way of stumbling through life. I was addicted, and little did I know then, I was on my way to destroying my life. I had been a good student and athlete. I went from hanging with the "brainy" kids and athletes, to hanging with drug dealers and gang bangers. Because, in order to feed my new found addiction to weed and alcohol, I needed to run with the crowd that could provide what I "needed." By the time I was 14, I was well into my addiction. I still went to school, but only for the weed and the girls. My grandmother and I were smoking, together, regularly. I would bring a joint, and she would bring a joint.

My mother had experienced a mental breakdown when I was 9. She would be in and out of mental institutions all the time. Ironically, her mental breakdown was caused by a troubled marriage to a heroin addict. When I was 15 my dear friend [name of friend] was murdered and my life changed. I began hanging with mostly gang bangers. I started smoking PCP, or as we call it sherm. Named after the Sherman stick we dipped in PCP/angel dust, and then smoked. I went from using depressants to using hallucinogens.

Now comes the criminal element of my addiction. I sporadically attended school, played sports, and gangbanged, but I was always high. I became a full time gang banger and criminal, when my grandmother kicked me out of her home for wrecking my grandfather's car. I was so high off the sherm and alcohol at the time of the accident, I was afraid to use PCP after that, so I quit. So, I started smoking weed more than ever. I was high all day, everyday between the ages of 16 and 18. I was able to pay for my weed and alcohol habit with the money I got from my various criminal activities, such as home invasions, commercial burglaries, robberies, and cocaine sales.

In the 1980s [name of city] was a haven for cocaine and crack. I was exposed to the "Dope Boy" life through one of my uncles; he had been a hustler and alcoholic all of my life. Without knowing it, somewhere deep inside of me, I aspired to be just like him. My world became chaotic, and I liked it. I became a full fledged criminal, gang banger, and addict. My mentality had become "fuck school and my family." I was a full time thug and addict, I didn't need anything but those two things in my life. I dabbled in coke/crack, smoked a few primos, or weed blunts mixed with coke. I even tried snorting a little coke. I never really liked the coke high, I was already a fast talking, fast moving person, and the coke just amplified these attributes. Plus, getting high on coke was frowned upon by the homies. To them smoking coke in any way made you a dope fiend. So, I reverted back to smoking weed and drinking daily. I stayed in a daze for about two and a half years, and then I caught my first case. First degree murder, at 18½ years of age. That case was dropped after seventy- two hours, due to the lack of evidence. It was a blessing, but a curse at the same time. With that case being dropped I thought I could do anything and get away with it. Then I started doing acid with this white girl I had met, and soon moved onto mushrooms. I caught another case at 19, this time it was a drug case, followed by a plethora of cases, all in a row.

Out of the next twenty years, I would spend twelve of them locked up. It took me a couple of years to figure out that there was a direct correlation between my getting high, drunk, and going to jail. The way I figured it, if I just smoked weed and drank, I wasn't an addict. I wasn't what would have been considered a dope fiend by my homies or myself for that matter. In 1998, while in prison, I met [names of treatment providers]. Finally, I'd met some people that would help me understand about my drug and alcohol addiction. And they did so without turning their backs on me and leaving me without the tools I needed to combat my disease of addiction. It was through a prison program called [name of program] and the help of [name of treatment providers] of the [name of treatment center], that my life changed. I no longer think of drugs and alcohol the same, thanks to them. My life will be forever changed. [name of treatment provider] was my counselor and [name of treatment provider] was the director of the program. [name of treatment provider] saved my butt and allowed me to graduate, despite myself.

I learned that drug and alcohol addiction is an incurable disease. If you are an addict, you're an addict for life. The beauty of recovery, for me, is that it's a choice. Anyone can choose to use drugs or alcohol, or choose not to use drugs or alcohol. I have come to realize that drug and alcohol addiction can be avoided. It is through experience and continuous trial and failure that I realize that I can not use, no matter what. I cannot take that first drink, I cannot take that first toke of anything, because, for me, drug and alcohol use lead to criminal behaviors. Which, in turn, lead to prison. I get drunk, I break the law, and get caught. If I get high, I break the law, and get caught. I now fully understand that I cannot use, because my thinking goes astray from the norm. I will not destroy myself or my life again. I am my best ally and my worst enemy. I look at the person in the mirror, who had been blessed with so much, but achieved so little. I used to blame everyone for my problems, except for myself. First, it was because I didn't know my father. Then it was because of the hood I grew up in and the family I had. And let's not forget the "white man," yes I used that copout too. I now realize that although the government has prisons and the criminal justice system is designed to punish and destroy, then rehabilitate, it is not the "white man's" fault that I smoke weed and PCP, or that I bought liquor, got drunk and did extremely stupid things. Those were all my decisions, I was never forced to get high or drunk. It was my choice and my choice alone.

I have come to realize that the quality of my life is determined by the choices I make. I have no more chances with the justice system. I now have several felonies, I have been in both state and federal prisons. My new "free" life is determined by my actions and choices. I am going to do everything in my power to stay clean and sober. I will no longer partake in any illegal activities, no matter what. Meaning, I cannot and will not drink alcohol or smoke weed, because, as I mentioned before, I break the law when I do these things.

During my time of going in and out of jail and the streets I was blessed with two beautiful, wonderful children, first a daughter and then a son. My children need their father to stay clean and sober, their futures rely on it.

After the [name of the program] I thought I had all of the necessary tools to stay clean and sober. Most of all, freedom from crime, prison, or any form of incarceration. I started attending AA and NA regularly, and went back to school. I even started working full time, for the first time in my life. I even met a wonderful, beautiful girl and had a handsome son, my life was going great. I stayed clean and sober for three years. I decided to celebrate my success. I drank a bottle of champagne for New Years. I drank that bottle and the old monster of addiction came roaring back at me and once again my life was destroyed.

I started drinking once a week, then smoking once a week. This led to the destruction of my "free" life. And my wonderful, beautiful female and I started arguing, because I started cheating and hanging out on the streets, instead of being home with my family. She and I split and I moved on my own. I graduated from the community college I attended, with an A.A. in mental health. Two months after graduation I was back to using, and had completely separated from my family. I wasn't calling my daughter that often and was back on the road to self destruction, once again. I started using daily, and had moved in with two females. I found myself in the midst of constant chaos and mischief, just how I used to like it. One thing led to another and I caught another case, this time landing me in the Federal System.

All of the hard work and effort almost went down the drain, thankfully, my three years plus of sobriety paid off. I was able to depend on solid, legitimate people for bail, legal, and mental support. Although I was immersed into my old criminal behavior I allowed God to guide me to the right kind of people. I developed and maintained a friendship with my sponsor. I made a real connection with my children, both my daughter and son. I was able to, not only be in my children's lives, but I was fully participating in my son's everyday life. With the drugs and alcohol in my life I was unable to do that. I am thankful to God, "The Creator of All Things," for blessing me with life and allowing me to experience freedom, sanity, peace, and happiness. Although I was sent to Federal Prison for fifty-one months, I am a better man. I will not fail, mainly because I will not relapse, no matter what. My life is on the line, I cannot go back to prison, because my horrendous past, I would surely get life, no breaks for me.

My daughter is now 17 and my son is 7, both need their father. I will sacrifice everything to achieve and keep my freedom. Alcohol and drugs are out of my life. I am an alcoholic and addict, I now know and understand this. I am also a father and a good student, I have received 9 credits to achieve a B.A. in general studies and drug and alcohol counseling. I would destroy everything I've obtained if I go back to getting high or drunk. Sober is the only way for me to stay free. Being sober is allowing me to be the best me I can be.

Anyone that believes that drugs or alcohol is not addictive is fooling themselves. I know not everyone is an addict or alcoholic. For me, I destroyed my dreams by using and breaking the law. If God saw fit to give me a second chance, I am going to take full advantage of it. If a person is blessed with life, health, and freedom make the most of it.

There's an old Chinese Proverb that states "a journey of a thousand steps begins with one." How true that is, I am on that journey, through sobriety. I live sober, no longer actively participating in gang life, criminal activity, and most importantly drugs or alcohol.

I feel as though I can become and achieve anything I choose to become or achieve. I have been blessed with outstanding health, both mentally and physically, and I plan on taking full advantage of this new life I've been given. I will move and groove to the rhythms of life, on life's terms, no longer trying to dull or enhance reality. I can now see and think clearly and life is great! Life is great because I am alive, free, and sober.

Never again will I take it for granted, I will cherish and appreciate every moment.

Analysis of Rick

Unfortunately, Rick ended up back in prison after writing this. He is now in a half-way house. According to someone who has worked with Rick for 10 years, "The problem with [his] self-report . . . is the lies and half-truths." (I can't provide the source for the quote because it would violate confidentiality, but it was a personal correspondence from someone whose opinion I trust). So, Rick doesn't go into much detail on what he refers to as "mischief," but it is all criminal activity and other socially inappropriate behavior. You don't have to read very far between the lines to see that he would easily meet the criteria for ASPD.

I don't want to downplay the impact of Rick's childhood environment. It certainly sounds difficult, with a single mother in the inner city with alcoholism and drug addiction in the adults around him. However, his mother was a professional with a steady job as a teacher. He doesn't give us much detail about his mother's "mental breakdown," the heroin addict she was married to, or who raised him while his mother was "in and out of mental institutions." If it was his grandmother who he smoked marijuana with, that was certainly a problem. So, if Rick is telling the truth, he had a difficult childhood and his gravitation to gangs and drug use is understandable.

This is not a sociology book. I certainly believe that the environment a child is raised is significantly contributes to how he or she turns out. But, some kids survive an environment like Rick's and some don't. At the point that the person can be diagnosed with ASPD, it probably doesn't matter what caused it. We just know if it is very difficult to change.

Rick focuses on his addiction to alcohol and other drugs and leaves a lot of details out about his antisocial activities. He tells us that as an adolescent he participated in "home invasions, commercial burglaries, robberies, and cocaine sales" and was arrested for murder when he was 18. Rick spent 12 of the next 20 years incarcerated. I believe that Rick is an addict, with most of his drug use involving alcohol and marijuana. I also think Rick is an ASPD criminal. He wasn't committing crimes to simply support his alcohol and other drug use. He may have been under the influence of drugs while he was committing criminal acts, but he did what he did because he is an addict with ASPD who engages in criminal behavior. The language of "I caught another case" sounds like some random event occurred. Rick committed a crime and got caught.

The language of recovery and redemption was similar to what he heard from Henry. With Rick, it is more obvious that these are just words he uses for effect and not concepts that he has internalized. With many ASPD patients, treatment providers and law-enforcement personnel hear these utterances because the ASPD patient quickly learns that this is a way to escape unpleasant consequences (e.g., incarceration). After a few relapses and criminal acts, it becomes clear that the addict with ASPD is just saying what he or she knows everyone wants to hear. Rick is a great example of this.

CONCLUSION

The two case examples in this chapter showed that although patients with ASPD are very difficult to manage, there is some hope for long-term sobriety and avoidance of the criminal justice system for some of them. It may be that those with ASPD who are not impulsive and aggressive have a better prognosis that those who are. The contrast between Henry and Rick provides some anecdotal evidence for this possibility.

The more important issue involves the impact of ASPD patients in the addiction-treatment process. Both Henry and Rick became engaged in treatment while in the criminal justice system. This seems appropriate. As we learned in the first part of the chapter, the proportion of ASPD individuals in the criminal justice system is quite high. We can be confident that Henry and Rick were among many other ASPD patients while in the prison treatment system. Because treatment was conducted within the prison system, it was quite appropriate to implement procedures that would be most effective with ASPD patients. That is, random drug testing, withdrawal of privileges for noncompliance, and punishment for inappropriate behavior could be easily made part of the treatment system. A disruptive individual or someone who came up "dirty" on a drug screening could simply be expelled from the treatment program and returned to the general prison population. Of course, those ASPD patients who are the most manipulative and intelligent could easily learn what to say and how to act to avoid any negative consequences. But, regardless of how they get there, it is the desired outcome. Whether or not Henry really believes all the recovery and redemption stuff he tells in his story is not really relevant. As long as he acts lawfully, stays sober, and generally acts appropriately, we have to be satisfied with that outcome. Henry may still manipulate others and have little ability to connect with people in any meaningful manner. There is really nothing that any therapist, social worker, sponsor, or clergyperson can do about that.

Outside the criminal justice setting, there is some concern about ASPD patients and non-ASPD patients being part of the same treatment groups. There is little likelihood that ASPD patients can be managed effectively in these settings, because the rapid implementation of severe consequences for inappropriate behavior is usually not possible in non-correctional settings. If ASPD patients are in non-institutional treatment as part of sanctions imposed by the criminal justice system, there is some leverage, but the bureaucratic process can be a problem. For example, an ASPD patient is ordered to outpatient treatment as an alternative to prison. The patient misses group and is disruptive when he is present. The therapist has to contact the appropriate law enforcement professional and that individual has to contact the patient. Sometimes the therapist has to wait for the next court date for the patient to be punished. These delays are not helpful with ASPD patients, who must experience immediate, significant consequences if there is any hope to modify their behavior.

It is also possible that ASPD patients have a detrimental impact on the treatment process for non-ASPD patients. If ASPD patients are disruptive, abusive, and/or noncompliant, it occupies the time of the treatment providers and the resources of the treatment facilities. In such instances, non-ASPD patients receive less attention. Thus, it may be necessary to make efforts to treat ASPD patients with substance use disorders separately from other patients with substance use disorders. This will be discussed in more detail in the final chapter.

FOUR

Functional Addicts

INTRODUCTION

The largest subtype, the functional addict, is quite a mystery. There is very little research available on functional addicts, primarily because members of this group so rarely come to the attention of treatment providers or other clinicians (at least for alcohol or other drug problems). By the very definition of the group, functional addicts are maintaining jobs and relationships, managing to avoid the criminal justice system, and are not experiencing serious health problems. Although functional addicts may have had problems in any or all of these areas at some point, these problems did not result in treatment for their alcohol or other drug use. It may be that the life problems were not associated with substance abuse, the problems were not serious enough to result in some form of intervention, or the functional addict adapted his or her behavior to avoid these problems in the future. For example, a functional addict who received a DUI in early adulthood may avoid drinking and driving in the future.

There are also other possible explanations to explain how functional addicts avoid treatment. As will be seen in the three case examples, functional addicts do not seem to experience the same serious consequences of their alcohol and other drug use as we saw with disease model and ASPD addicts. For some reason, functional addicts may not progress in their alcohol and other drug use as rapidly as other addicts. Although this is simply my own clinical observation and is not based on scientific research, it seems to me that the functional addicts I have encountered have a very high tolerance for alcohol and other drugs, and they do not seem to lose the ability to behave within the broad range of "normal" even when under the influence of alcohol or other drugs. In contrast to many other addicts, functional addicts under the influence of drugs and alcohol do not seem to have personality changes, to lose control of their emotions, or to suffer blackouts. Therefore, while other addicts may be visibly intoxicated; become obnoxious, belligerent, or morose; or engage in inappropriate behavior, functional addicts are generally behaving just as they normally do when sober. They may be more social, humorous, or subdued, but not to the extent that it generates irritation or concern from others. Furthermore, I have noticed that functional addicts refrain from using alcohol and other drugs in clearly inappropriate settings or at inappropriate times (e.g., during the work day). In other words, functional addicts seem to be able to exert more control over their use than other addicts.

There may be one other factor that distinguishes some functional addicts from other types of addicts: luck. As you will see in the examples in this chapter, these functional addicts have engaged in alcohol and other drug use in some risky situations. They just escaped the consequences.

CASE EXAMPLES

Interview with George

George is a 60-year-old retired school administrator. He is married to his second wife, who continues to work for herself in a service industry. George has two adult children and one grandchild. He has a cordial relationship with them. His wife does not have biological children. The relationship between George and his wife has been very strained for some time, and they basically lead separate lives but continue to live together. George spends his time reading, mostly nonfiction books on current events, philosophy, and religion and on outdoor activities such as biking and snowboarding. He readily admits to preferring to be alone and is very cynical about people and society. George maintains some social relationships that involve his outdoor activities but has no close friendships. When he was working, George was well liked, fairly successful, and seen as having a very good sense of humor. However, he occasionally had some problems with making inappropriate comments to female workers.

Interviewer (I):   Tell me about the first time you used alcohol and other drugs

George (G):   I really can't remember my first experience with alcohol. As far back as I can remember, both my parents drank. My first experience with marijuana was seventh grade. Some friends had it, we went to some motel on [name of street] and it was the first time I ever smoked marijuana. I kind of liked it. It wasn't something I could get frequently at that time. It was hard to get. That was the beginning. Once I got into high school, it was drinking beer, anything we could get actually, but I always enjoyed marijuana more than alcohol. In those days, it was like—god, I'm just trying to remember—$10 to $20 bags. Seeds and stems.

I: By the time you started high school, how often were you smoking?

G: Maybe once or twice a week.

I: What about drinking?

G: Every weekend.

I: When you were in high school, did you try anything else besides alcohol and marijuana?

G: No, [name of city] at that time, at least the people I was around, no one talked about hard drugs like heroin or cocaine or even acid. I never saw anything like that in high school, which was 1965 to 1968. [Name of city] was really small then. Didn't see stuff like that. Heard about stuff like that, but never saw it. Then I joined the Marine Corps after high school. Of course, while I was stateside in the Marine Corps, I didn't smoke marijuana, but once I got to Vietnam, after everyone became comfortable with you being the new person in the unit, and they would speak more freely, I realized there were some people who smoked dope. I became friends with them.

I: Where did you get it?

G: In the villages. You'd go out in the village and, for example, [for] a carton of Kool cigarettes, you could get 100 joints. Rolled and put in plastic. I'm sure the money went to the North Vietnamese or the Viet Cong but it was very similar if you've seen the movie *Platoon*. It was very similar to that in that there was a very distinct group of people who either smoked dope and drank. Since you weren't 21, technically you couldn't buy alcohol where I was in Vietnam. When we came back out of the field, I would hang out with the people who smoked dope and I would smoke for a day or two and then they would round us all back up and we could go back out in the field. The boozers all got drunk and we would meet up and go do our thing. It was always done when we came back out of the field and nobody smoked when you were out on patrol or anything like that. Everyone kept their shit together. Once you came to a built-up area to rest, everyone rested in their own way, so that was very common.

I: Did you see heroin use by guys there?

G: No, no needles, none of that. In the rear areas, there were. You could get it easily. But out in the field, no. It was basically beer but it was not refrigerated, so typically, any beer you drank was warm. For every day you were in the field, you got one can of beer. And, they would bring you back and have a big party. Kind of crazy. Real crazy. So, then what happened? I had three more months in the Marine Corps.

I: How long were you in Vietnam?

G: 13 months. I had three more months in the Marine Corps so I signed up to stay three more months in Vietnam because I didn't want to come home.

I: You stayed 3 more months in Vietnam?

G: I didn't want to come home and be a stateside Marine with a shaved head. Staying in Vietnam was scary but I thought it would be a better thing to do. So I signed up for the three more months to stay. I hadn't seen a friend in a long time. He came back out of the field. We were sitting in a tent, smoking a joint, and an officer came in and caught us. We kept on smoking the joint. He came back with some other officers and, it's not like you are really arrested, what happened was they took me to my commanding officer and my CO gave orders to send me home. So, that's what they did.

I: But everybody was doing it, right? Why did they send you home?

G: They just didn't want me there. All these officers saw me smoking with this guy and they wanted me out [of] there, so they sent me home. That's what happened. There was a time when I liked psychedelics. When I came back home to Camp Pendleton, every payday all of us Marines went off base.

I: Can I stop you a moment. You said you liked psychedelics. When. . . .

G: After Vietnam. After I came back home and I was at Camp Pendleton for three months, there were some Marines there who had contacts, could get some LSD. I started experimenting with that; kind of liked it for a while. Enjoyed it. Maybe, I would say I probably did it about 50 times. After a while, it just became something I didn't like to do anymore. The interesting thing to me is that I have always been someone who has been pretty disciplined. And so, I don't like something I totally lose control [over]. As crazy as this sounds, I liked to cash checks on LSD, drive, go to weird places to see if I would get freaked out. Never really did. I was always able to kind of keep it together. I never had flashbacks or bad trips. To me, it was all just kind of fun. Nothing bad really happened to me mentally, or car accidents, or anything like that. So, then what happened after that? After the Marine Corps, I came back to [name of city]. I had sent some stuff back from Vietnam. When you first got to Vietnam, you could mail anything home, anything. Grenades, anything. And you didn't have to have anybody sign for it. Before I left, if you had a package that was large, you had to open it and show it to your sergeant. And he'd have to sign and you had to package it up. But before that happened, I probably sent back 100 joints in letters to my girlfriend and some of my friends and they kept them for me. So, when I came home, I sat around and smoked for probably 2 to 3 months.

I: How old were you then?

G: Probably 20 to 21 years old. Somewhere in there. I was working at the [name of place]. I had been working there before I went into the Marine Corps as a shuttle-bus driver. So when I got back from the war, I got a job there again as a maintenance man at this motel. One day, they started building a chain-link enclosure in the basement of the parking garage and I asked my boss what that was going to be for, and he said it was going to be for guest's dogs and that one of my jobs was going to be to go in there and scoop up the poop. And it was that day that I walked back up to the university and filled out the paperwork to enroll.

I: Didn't you tell me about some story when you were stateside where you got busted coming back into camp?

G: Yeah, yes, that did happen. When I was still at Camp Pendleton and on paydays we would go off the base and buy a bag of dope or whatever somebody wanted to buy. They always had four gates to get back into the base and we knew one of those gates would have dogs and they would spend more time looking in your car and seeing if you were OK. It was kind of a game of cops and robbers, of choosing which gate to go back in. One night, I chose the wrong gate and we had been smoking dope and I had taken some LSD, and they took me out of the car. It was the first time I really ever lost it. They asked me my serial number, which of course every Marine is supposed to remember, and I still remember to this day but that day when I was on marijuana and the acid I couldn't spit it out fast enough. So, they ended up tearing my car apart and they found one hit of acid. For the three months I was at Camp Pendleton, they always held it over my head. "We are going to send you to Fort Leavenworth. We're going to prosecute your ass." Well, come to find out when my last day came, I had to go to all these different places on the base to sign out of the Marine Corps. When I went to the legal department, they said there was this hold on my records, and this sergeant major, this high-ranking enlisted man said, "What happened to you, Marine?" I said, "Well,

I picked up some hitchhiker, they said they found this hit of acid that must have fallen out of his pocket." He said, "That's a bunch of bullshit. Just sign my papers." I was so happy. I said, "Cool." I signed the papers and left. So, I dodged that bullet. I also had a time when I first came home from the war and got a job working in [name of city] on the [name of transportation system]. Didn't really use any drugs there. I drank. But no drugs. That was maybe a two-year period. When I moved back to [name of city], I met up with some friends and basically from that time, from the time I was 22, I've smoked marijuana ever since with hardly any periods in between. There some periods in there I never drank too. I've gone through periods of doing that. I've smoked marijuana ever since. It's never really affected me I think. I'm disciplined. When I had tests or things I had to do. I never smoked during the day or anything like that. I always, I don't know, keep your shit together. That's what's always driven me. Important to me to do a good job and do things correctly, so I wouldn't want to put myself at risk to do that during the day and get caught, something like that. That's never been a problem for me. Or drinking. Just something I've never done. When I was working.

I: So from the time you were 22 . . .

G: I've smoked marijuana every day.

I: So, was there ever a time, can you think of any time when there was a consequence, or something you avoided, or were pulled over by the police, anything like that?

G: There was a time when I was moving back from [name of city], I was pulled over by the highway patrol outside [name of city] and they looked into an ashtray that was in my dad's truck and there was a 16mm film canister, and he asked me what was in it and I said, "I don't know." There was actually a few flakes of marijuana and he poked his nose in it and said, "That's marijuana," and he gave it back to me and said, "Where are you going?" I said I was going to [name of city]. He said, "Get the hell out of here." That's close to a consequence. I've taken risks sometimes going on snowboard trips to [name of place] or [name of place] where I've packed my snowboard bag with marijuana, which has made me very nervous, but nothing has ever happened. Two years ago on a fishing trip I was pulled over by the highway patrol for speeding and, this is amazing, there were three of us in the truck—this is a great story. Three of us in the truck. We had stopped to get a beer. We were on a stretch of highway where you sometimes drive for hours and see no one. And, I'm going down this highway and I had smoked a bowl. I was driving the truck.

The other two guys don't smoke marijuana. It's kind of rolling in there and my radar detector went off just as this other car came over the rise, this highway patrolman. Anyway, he pulls me over. He can barely see into the truck. He's a really short dude and my truck sits up high. Short guy. He starts giving me crap about my radar detector. "See, that radar detector didn't help you." And he never asked for my driver's license. We had to hand the beers back to the guy behind me and I had smoked marijuana in the car and he goes, "Do you know how fast you were going?" And I go, "I know I was going over the speed limit." He says, "You were going 97." "Oh, OK." He never looked in the car. We had loaded guns, we had dope, we had beer, open cans of beer. That was kind of freaky, just by chance. Typically, I usually never smoke marijuana in my car. Now days. I usually don't do that. That day I was on a fishing trip in the middle of nowhere. I thought it was OK. I kept my shit together. It's funny. He never even asked me for my driver's license. Officer Black. Eventually, he says, "Where you guys going?" "We're going fishing." "You guys going to [name] Creek?" He gave me shit about my radar detector. It was amazing. That's it. Over the years, I had ski patrol at [name of place]. We were standing in the middle of a run smoking a joint. He came up behind us, "You guys shouldn't be doing that here." Ski patrol usually don't say anything. Up there at [name of ski resort], kind of back of the mountain, there is this huge cave, you can, any day, ski into there and there is a hodge podge of skiers and boarders smoking. Passing joints around. Over the years, sitting on lifts, someone will say, "You don't mind if I fire up, do you?" "You want to smoke a bowl with me, or are you cool?" It's pretty common. I wonder. You read statistics about how many ghost marijuana smokers there are and I think it's much bigger that we admit to. Can they measure that by how big the marijuana crop is? I don't think people tell the truth. The only person I've actually told is my doctor. But, that wasn't a big deal. Even [name of person], just before she was going through radiation, I was sitting with her and the doctor says, you use any kind of drugs? "Well, I smoke marijuana." For [name of person], her doctor prescribed a medication , forget the name of it, it was for nausea. It was $100 a pill. And we actually got the insurance company to pay for it. [name of person] smoked through all those sessions and it seemed to help. She did take the $100 pills, but the marijuana seemed to help. She still smokes. She likes to smoke before she goes to bed. I don't know. When I think of the work I do as a [name of job] working with kids who get in trouble with marijuana, sometimes I felt a little out of sorts when I had to deal with that.

I: Out of sorts? What do you mean?

G: Hypocritical. Here I am someone who smokes dope basically once a day and here I am with this kid. I tried to rationale it the best I could but . . . I don't know.

I: Have you had any health problems as a result?

G: No.

I: Did you ever go through a period of time where you thought, "Gee, I need to stop doing this"?

G: Well, when I say I smoked every day, there have been times where I didn't have the money or I might go 2 or 3 weeks without doing it. Not a problem. Not that I don't think, "Gee, it would be nice to smoke one." But it's not that big of [a] deal. Then I think, if it's not that big of [a]deal, why do you do it? But, it is something I enjoy. I look at the people I'm around athletically and it is funny. I'm a little hyperactive. Multi-tasker. Most of the people that I know in sports activities describe themselves that way too. I've noticed that. And the risk, adrenaline junkie sort of deal. I have a little bit of that in me and I don't know if that helps calm me down. I don't know, it seems to attract a lot of people with that kind of makeup. That I have noticed. Like the learning disabled population. In a sense, they like it. I don't know. Hasn't really affected me. If I was doing something that would put me in jail or I'd lose my money, my family, or my children, I wouldn't take the risk. But this has never been something like that. At least, I've never seen it that way. In my life.

I: What about other drugs? Cocaine, ever tried that?

G: A few times. I never really liked it. I don't like to be speeded up. I'm a little antsy anyway. I don't like that kind of buzzing. I did when I was in college take some cross tops, methamphetamines, to stay up and study, but never enjoyed that because the come down, you are grinding your teeth, never enjoyed the come down. So, that's not something I like.

I: Prescription drugs?

G: Never. I don't like pills. Pills kind of scare me. I don't like taking pills. I think a couple of times I was in high school I may have taken some black beauties and some Seconal, reds I think they called them, but I never liked them either. Pills are scary. I don't know if that makes sense in that marijuana is a plant and it doesn't seem like it is going to hurt you. Another rationalization perhaps [laughs]. It's funny. We have friends. If I'm over at their house and they aren't smokers and I want to take a puff, I just go into my room and puff and come back. I'd much rather smoke a bunch of marijuana than drink alcohol and be hung over and sick to my stomach and all that. Marijuana has never done that to me. It has always been kind of mellow and I like it. I don't know. At 60 years old, I think, gosh George, when are you going to stop being a kid? I have probably been buying dope here from the same guy for probably 10 years, and I've never really talked to gramps about the nature of his clientele but he has told me, "You wouldn't believe the number of teachers." I never ask, don't want to go there, but it is always amazing to me. In fact, I met a friend of [name of someone's] mother, a guy, younger than me, a friend of the family. I'm up in the trees at [name of place] smoking a joint and he skis up to me and takes a puff. Blew me away. I mean, I had no idea. This guy worked for [name of company], big muckety-muck position. Whoa, yeah, one for the team. Maybe we should have marijuana Olympics. I have a marijuana T-shirt. I'm ready to get a marijuana baseball cap. At this point, who cares? It's kind of silly. What else do you want to know? There was a point in my first marriage where I had to be a little private about it. My first wife, although she never put her foot down, she just didn't like it. More in the sense she just frowned on it. She never really tried to stop me. I just wouldn't rub her nose in it. I went out with the guys and got high. Or, if I had to go someplace, I'd go out for a ride in the car and come back. Other than that, when I got remarried, since marijuana was a part of my life, I guess, I had to be sure I was going to be with someone who was OK with it. That's how society looks at people who smoke marijuana. You are a loser and a burnout. You're never going to make much of yourself. I think there are probably more people strung out on alcohol than are strung out on marijuana or who are losers. It doesn't make you violent—at least it doesn't make me. In that sense. Just racing to the plate of brownies [laughs].

Analysis of George

Because George's primary drug of choice is marijuana, it would be useful to briefly discuss marijuana as a drug of abuse. Disconnecting the problems resulting from the drug from marijuana's legal status can be challenging for some people. In this discussion, the legal status of a drug is irrelevant. If George smoked a little marijuana in the evening to relax the same way many adults use alcohol, a description of George as a "functional addict" would be inappropriate. With regard to any illicit drug or alcohol, we are only concerned about the problems associated with such use. However, if George was arrested for possession of marijuana, and he persisted in putting himself in situations where another arrest might occur, that would be considered a "problem" associated with marijuana use.

Many people believe that marijuana is a relatively harmless drug and that people do not develop an addiction to it. Separating the propaganda from the facts about marijuana is difficult for the general public. The federal government has tended to exaggerate or misrepresent dangers about marijuana and legalization proponents have minimized or denied any adverse effects. The fact is that any mind-altering drug can cause problems for some people. Compared to alcohol or other illicit drugs, marijuana is probably less harmful. However, any treatment provider can attest to cases where clients were dependent on marijuana. George may be correct that there are many "ghost" marijuana users, especially among those of us who grew up in the 1960s and 1970s, but nevertheless, marijuana is a drug that is abused.

Of the three functional addict cases, George's is the most dubious in terms of the label "addict." That said, George tends to minimize his use of marijuana and the consequences of his drug use (I can't divulge how I know this because it might compromise George's confidentiality).

Based on George's story and my knowledge of his situation, it would be difficult to diagnose George with a substance dependence disorder (the criteria for substance dependent disorders and substance abuse disorders were provided in Chapter 1). However, he would meet the criteria for a substance abuse disorder because he frequently drives while under the influence of marijuana, and that would constitute "recurrent substance use in situations in which it is physically hazardous," which is one of the criteria for a substance abuse disorder. Only one of the four criteria is necessary for a diagnosis.

It is clear from George's story how the element of "luck" impacts how serious the drug problem is perceived. There were examples from George's military history that certainly could have resulted in more serious consequences than actually occurred. George also related two examples of contact with police officers where he could have been arrested. In the most recent episode, George was under the influence of marijuana while driving a car at high speed, there were open bottles of alcohol in the car, and there were loaded weapons. Imagine what would have happened if George had been involved in a serious traffic accident. There would have been no doubt in anyone's mind that George had a drug problem. Not only was he driving under the influence of an intoxicating substance but his judgment was seriously impaired to allow alcohol and loaded weapons in his car. The fact that no serious consequences occurred was George's good fortune, which included an unobservant police officer.

George has become increasingly isolated, antisocial, and cynical over time. Again, I can't divulge how I know this. It is impossible to state definitively whether this is related to his use of marijuana. It is very likely that there is a cyclical nature to George's isolation and marijuana use. Because George worked in a stressful situation in the public schools for many years, he developed a negative view about human behavior. Marijuana was a stress relief and a way of distancing himself from normal interactions with people, who he generally found to be disappointing. In retirement, he is able to avoid nearly all contact with people he finds distasteful. Smoking marijuana helps him to focus on his own thoughts and beliefs, which are the only ones he finds "normal." Since George is unable to find many kindred souls, he retreats into books and marijuana for the only companionship he finds satisfying.

In helping students conceptualize addiction, I often use the analogy of intimate partners. For an addict, the monogamous intimate relationship is with alcohol or other drugs. George exemplifies a person who has an intimate relationship with marijuana. This relationship provides the companionship and validation he needs. It is monogamous because he has no other intimate relationships.

Mark's Story

Mark is a 58-year-old man. He has been in a committed relationship for more than 10 years and has been married twice before. Mark has adult children and several grandchildren and is close to all of them. He has held a professional position for more than 25 years. Mark has never been arrested and has no serious medical conditions. This story was told to the interviewer in person, but the only question was, "What alcohol and drugs have you done today?" Mark told the rest without interruption.

Today? Let's see, I took three tramadol [Ultram], one at 8, one at 10, and one at 12. At 2, I had half a cup of coffee and half a cup of Baileys. At 3:30, I had one puff on my marijuana pipe, just enough to get a buzz. At 4 and 5, I had a beer. Then, I stopped because Kathy [not her real name] was coming home at about 7:30 and I needed to be pretty sober by the time she got home. She knows about the pills (she handed them out to me in the morning). But, she would not like the alcohol and marijuana.

I don't normally drink, especially not in the afternoon on a workday. But, I have been taking six to seven pain pills a day (Loratabs and Ultram, or lories and ulties as we call them). Today was the first day in a long time that I had cut down to three and I was feeling a little antsy. Also, I knew Kathy would be home later than usual, so I had time to indulge.

OK. You want me to start at the beginning, right? Before I start, I just want to say that I don't want anyone to get the idea that I'm proud of what

I am going to tell you. I wish I wasn't like this, you know, using drugs all the time. Every day, I think about how I can cut down or stop. I know it isn't healthy or productive and I feel like a hypocrite. Given my position and what I've accomplished, I know it would shock a lot of people if they knew the drugs I take every day. I hope that never happens but it certainly could.

I remember the first time I drank alcohol very clearly. I was about 13 and my parents were out of town. I have one older brother and I don't remember where he was but I was home alone. I decided to see what everyone was so excited about. Both my parents drank regularly so there was a wide variety of alcohol around. Since the time I was little, I would get sips of my dad's beer so I knew what that tasted like. But, I don't think I had ever tasted any hard liquor. I can't remember what I started with but I think it was some kind of bourbon. It tasted really awful so I put some kind of soda pop in it. Then, I just started trying other stuff. We had gin and vodka and I drank them with soda. I remember being really surprised with how bad all this stuff tasted. And, I didn't really feel much of anything. Looking back, I guess I have a natural high tolerance for alcohol. But, after a while, I started to feel sick. I lay down on the couch in the living room. You know, that is one of the worst feelings in the world. You can't close your eyes because the room starts spinning and you can't keep them open because of the nausea. Anyway, I finally vomited all over the living room rug. Just when I finished, the phone rang and it was my mother checking up on me. This was the first time of the many times that I had to pretend to be normal when I wasn't. Although she thought something was wrong, I was able to convince her that everything was fine. I got off the phone and cleaned up the puke. I can't remember what happened after that.

It's really funny but you would think that a negative experience like this would keep a person from drinking for a very long time. I had a similar experience the first time I smoked. I stole a cigarette from the woman who cleaned our house and smoked it in the basement. It made me nauseous but I kept trying and eventually started smoking. I quit about 25 years ago but I guess that isn't what we are here for.

Anyway, I didn't start drinking regularly until high school, which was 10th grade in those days. So, I was around 16. I had a beer occasionally before then but the puking incident kept me from drinking anything else. When I was 14, my mother made me go to a party I didn't want to go to. We are Jewish and we called these parties "Jew parties" because they involved nerdy, religious Jewish families with kids I didn't hang out with. There was one other kid I hung out with there and I stole a beer from the refrigerator and he and I ditched the party. We were walking on the street and got picked up by plainclothes cops. I didn't have the beer by then but smelled like it. Also, I had cigarettes and firecrackers. They took me home. My dad was so shocked. I can still remember his face when we got to the door and the cops told him what happened. He just looked at me and said, "You???" I had never been in any serious trouble before then. Anyway, I had to go to juvenile court but just got a lecture. It did make me kind of famous among my peers. But, I was sincerely scared. I became much more sneaky and cautious after that.

OK. Let me move on to high school. I had been a pretty social, fairly popular kid in elementary school. In junior high, I was still social and popular but things changed. My parents were struggling in their business and their marriage (I found out later that my mother was having an affair), I turned into a skinny, ugly adolescent, and my school was pretty rough. While in my elementary school years, I thought the world was wonderful and everyone loved me, in junior high I started to see the dark side of life. So, in my sophomore year of high school (the first year, in the way our school system was structured), I started dating Denise, a girl who was kind of quiet and awkward too. We bonded to each other the way adolescents do out of the need for companionship and affection and to feel wanted. We were both good students and somewhat involved in school activities, and we became an inseparable couple. Although we certainly isolated ourselves, we still had some social life. There were parties where there was generally beer and I had a group of guys I played poker with. My parents owned a tavern (beer and wine) and they would supply us with beer for these gatherings. Now, I don't remember drinking any more than any of my other friends. Sometimes I would drink too much and get sick but so would everyone else. I remember hearing stories from acquaintances about how they would consume huge amounts of beer but I never did that. At one poker party, a guy who came to these events occasionally got pretty drunk. He had a motorcycle and started driving up and down our street at 2 in the morning. We couldn't reason with him. I was never like that. The only goofy thing I remember doing was climbing into the bath tub with all my clothes on with our dog. But, I can clearly remember the incident and knew I was being silly. There were a couple of jocks who came over once in a while who would become belligerent when they drank but my personality didn't really change when I was intoxicated. Back in those days, we didn't think much about drinking and driving and I know I drove many times after drinking. But, by the grace of God, no one had any accidents or serious injuries. My best friend did fall off a truck and got scraped up but was not seriously hurt. Oh, and he (my best friend) spent the night at his girlfriends house after one party. He had told his parents he was spending the night at my house. His father called at 7 in the morning asking for him. I was quite hung over and tried to cover for him. I had to jump in the car (no cell phones in those days) and drive a ½ hour to go wake him up. Other than those minor incidents, the only consequences I can remember were that the house smelled like vomit in the morning after these parties and I would have a hangover. But, that was about it.

Now, this was happening in the late 1960s so marijuana was starting to get popular with kids our age. But I never tried it. By our senior year, some of my friends were experimenting but Denise and I were spending so much time with each other that I wasn't really around it. I don't remember having any moral issues about pot but it just wasn't part of my environment.

One of the biggest regrets I have about my life is that I stayed in my hometown and went to the local university instead of going away to school. I had the grades and test scores to go elsewhere but I was too scared to venture out. Denise decided to go to a school about 90 miles from our hometown. I think it was her way of trying to distance herself from me but I wouldn't let her. I was miserable that first year and Denise eventually transferred back to my school after our sophomore year. A couple of my friends stayed home too. So, there were some people to hang out with. But, nothing really changed with regard to my alcohol use. In my junior year, a couple of friends and I got a house near campus and Denise lived right across the street with some other girls. One of my roommates was Denise's brother and he and I would often go out to a tavern at night, drink beer and play pinball. But, we didn't do anything too dramatic. We would share a pitcher of beer and then go home. Since I wasn't in a dorm or fraternity, there weren't any wild parties.

Denise and I got married before our senior year in college. She never really drank that much and I don't really remember drinking that much either. I may have had a beer or two at night but we were pretty poor so there weren't many nonessentials. After we graduated, she got a job as an elementary teacher and I went to graduate school in a field that I will not mention because it would give a clue about my identity. It was a field that led to a job after about 1½ years.

Graduate school really was a turning point in my life. I had never dated or even kissed any other girl but Denise. In graduate school, I was around smart, attractive women with the same interests as me. I was very attracted to these women but I was too uncertain about myself to do anything about it. Most of them were married anyway. We would see some of these couples socially and I was aware of how quiet and shy Denise was. I started to become aware of feeling unsatisfied with our relationship.

I know that some of this history doesn't seem to have much to do with my alcohol and drug use but, for me, it explains the life events that led me to start drinking more and to start using marijuana. I think that my alcohol use was pretty moderate for an extended period of time but escalated as I became more and more unhappy with Denise. By the way, I don't blame any of this on her. She was a great woman and actually blossomed personally and professionally after we divorced.

When I got my first job, Denise and I were, for the first time, financially secure and we bought a house. But, I was now surrounded by a lot of young women and I had a prestigious job (relatively speaking). I didn't think of myself as attractive but I did know how to use my knowledge and intelligence to impress people. (By the way, I don't want any of this to sound egotistical because I am painfully aware of my faults. But, I have gotten enough feedback over the years to know that I am smart, in an academic sense. I have also gotten enough feedback to know that I can be an asshole and that I'm manipulative.) So, I was getting a lot of attention from young, bright, attractive women. But I still didn't have the confidence to make any moves. I'd like to tell you it was because I had a moral value that did allow adultery but that would be delusional. I was just insecure and scared.

I still wasn't drinking a lot but even the little I did started to cause some problems between Denise and I. Her parents rarely drank and she wasn't used to regular alcohol use the way I was. I would almost always have a beer or two at dinner. Denise started to complain about this. I thought she was nuts. Honestly, I don't think I was drinking that much. But, I certainly had developed a high tolerance to alcohol and that was embarrassingly demonstrated at a dinner party. It was during my first year as a professional and one of my colleagues invited several couples over for dinner. The hosts were a bit older than Denise and I (we were 24) and they were much more sophisticated. When we arrived, they offered us cocktails and I had some kind of whisky. Now, the only time I drank hard liquor was at my parents. We didn't have it at our home. It was a good quality liquor as I recall and I drank pretty fast. As good hosts, they kept refilling my glass until they ran out of whatever it was that I was drinking. They got something else but I could see that they were at appalled at my intake. I didn't get drunk at all. To this day, I cringe when I think about that evening and what these people must have thought of me. Needless to say, that was the last social engagement we were invited to.

Then, Denise got pregnant. This was planned and I was thrilled. I love kids and really wanted my own. About two months into the pregnancy, Denise hurt her back. I don't remember what happened. She stayed pretty much incapacitated for the remainder of the pregnancy and about six months after our son was born. Our sex life, which was boring to begin with, was nonexistent during this time. Now, you might be saying that we just weren't very creative but Denise just would not do anything. She said every possible movement was too painful. So, I was abstinent for over a year. This was really a dark time. We were both miserable. I treated Denise like my patient. I did things for her but did them without kindness or affection. Both of our families lived close by so we did have help. Our only outings were to go to my parent's house for dinner. When we got in the house, I would head straight to their liquor cabinet and make myself a VO on the rocks. It was probably a triple. I just poured. I would have a couple of those, a beer or two, and brandy after dinner. Then, I'd drive home. All I can tell you is that I didn't get very drunk. No one ever asked me if I was OK to drive. I remember falling asleep briefly one time but fortunately woke up before we crashed.

I was introduced to marijuana when I started an affair with Cheryl. I guess I was 26 or 27. We worked together and her husband had told her that he didn't love her anymore. I had figured out that being a sensitive listener was a good way to have women pay attention to me so I became her confidant. That went on for several months. Although I was attracted to her, I didn't think she would be interested in me and I never did anything inappropriate with her. Along with another woman colleague, the three of us planned a weekend retreat at a nearby island. We all had personal crises going and needed to get away. I told Denise all about this (including my friendship with Cheryl) and she didn't object at all. By that time, our son had been born and Denise's sister agreed to stay with Cheryl while I was gone since Denise was still incapacitated with her back. Of course, looking back at this, I can see how much Denise and I were in denial. But, she seemed to have this blind trust in me; a belief that I would never betray her. Anyway, the other woman backed out of the trip and told us that we shouldn't go. Cheryl and this woman were friends and knew what was going to happen. But, Cheryl and I discussed it and decided that this other woman was silly. We were good friends and this was just going to be a time to relax and enjoy each other's company. What a bunch of bullshit. Then, Cheryl proposes that we stay in the same room to "save money." Of course, there would be two beds. I told Denise about this too and she said it was OK. Can you believe that? When we got to the room, guess what? There was only one bed. I can still picture Cheryl flopping down on that bed and smiling seductively at me and saying what a shame that was that there was only one bed. I was really flustered and said that we should ask them to bring in a roll-away bed. Anyway, we went to the bar and had some drinks (I drank beer) and dinner. There was a band and we slow danced. We kissed and I said, "I love my wife." Of course, that didn't stop us. We made love that night and that entire weekend. Now, I have to tell you: I didn't know what the fuck I was doing. Cheryl was my second lover and I knew absolutely nothing about pleasuring my partner. I don't think Denise had ever had an orgasm with me, nor did I even realize that she could or should. Cheryl must have been desperate or really liked me. As the affair progressed, she did teach me how to be a better lover and we developed a very passionate and satisfying sex life.

Sorry. I was supposed to talk about marijuana. Got distracted. Cheryl and I went on a backpacking trip for a couple of days, again with Denise's blessing. She didn't think anything was going on between Cheryl and me. Cheryl brought some pot and we smoked it. It was the first time I got high (I had a puff some months earlier with another friend but didn't feel anything). It was unbelievable. To this day, it is still the best high I have ever experienced. Sex was incredible. I remember feeling like my penis was enormous (it's not) and I was really loud. Cheryl had to tell me to be quiet because there were other campers in the area.

So, the affair went on for a while. Cheryl and I would drink brandy and smoke weed. Of course, affairs don't stay static and Cheryl and I were making a spectacle of ourselves. My brother (who worked in the same place I did) and my boss took me camping and tried to talk some sense into me. I remember my boss telling me to just fuck around but don't get attached. Good advice, huh? But, Cheryl and I had "fallen in love" and no one could dissuade me. Now, I was miserable. I was in love with another woman, had a child, was lying. Oh, I was also working and in school for my Ph.D. I was a bundle of anxiety. Denise and I actually had Cheryl over to the house for dinner and she spent the night. While my incapacitated wife was asleep in our bed, I was making out in the living room with Cheryl. Unfortunately for me, I do have a conscience so I was racked with guilt, but not enough to stop me.

I finally told Denise about the affair. Some deluded part of me thought that she would handle this information calmly, wish me good luck, and send me on my way to a life with Cheryl. It didn't quite happen that way. Denise freaked out, became hysterical, and pounded on me (she was small and still disabled so she couldn't do much damage). Over the next weeks, she became suicidal with an actual plan and a note. I was alarmed by her reaction and told Cheryl that we had to break it off.

Now, I know that all of this seems tangential to the subject of alcohol and drugs. But, all of this does lead to the next chapter in the drama that unleashed my alcohol and drug use. Denise and I sought out a marriage counselor. Unbeknownst to Denise, we went to the therapist who was treating Cheryl. Looking back, I know that this guy was as unethical as you can get. He was sleeping with many of this clients (including Cheryl). He suggested that Denise and I continue to live together but that we be allowed to do whatever we wanted without discussing it with each other. Of course, I thought this was great and, as you might expect, it wasn't long before Cheryl and I were at it again. Also, I felt free to drink as much as I wanted and smoke as much dope as I wanted. So, I was living in my house with Denise, taking care of my son, and living like a single guy. During this time, I had the only blackout I can remember. I went to some party with Cheryl, smoked weed and drank. The next day, I could not remember what happened between the time I left the party and I got home. No idea. I don't know why I had a blackout then and I have never had one since. But, it was freaky. Didn't slow me down though.

Eventually, Denise and I did divorce. I moved in with a guy I worked with and we had a blast. He introduced me to Stoli, a Russian vodka. We kept a bottle in the freezer. When I would get home from work, I would pour a glass of that stuff and just keep drinking it all night. I was also smoking dope but that was not a daily thing. With all of the disruption in my life, I put my doctoral program on hold. I was done with courses and just had to do my exams and my dissertation. After about a year, I changed jobs. So, I wasn't working with Cheryl anymore. She wanted a committed relationship and, with whatever little bit of sense I possessed, I realized that wouldn't be a good move for me. I liked the freedom too much. Eventually, Denise started dating someone who wanted what she did and she dumped me. I was upset but not enough to make any changes.

I began dating a woman (let's call her Wanda) at my new place of work. I wasn't crazy about her but she could drink me under the table. I had never had that experience before. Wanda lived about ½ hour from where I did. I would make myself a big glass of Stoli, get in the car, stop and buy a bottle of champagne, and go to Wanda's house. So, I'd drink on the way over and drink at her house. We smoked pot too but alcohol was definitely the primary drug. I remember going out with Wanda one night and after a movie or something, we went to a bar and started doing tequila shots. I had to stop after a while but Wanda kept on going. I was impressed. One day, I was supposed to go to her house for dinner but she didn't show up to work. I got a strange call from her telling me I could pick up the dinner at her house if I wanted to. I drove over in the middle of the day and found her drunk and suicidal. I took her to an emergency room and they admitted her to an alcohol treatment program. I participated in a lot of the family stuff and learned a lot about alcoholism. Of course,

I didn't identify with it; I thought of myself as a moderate drinker and Wanda actually reinforced that. She stayed sober (and I still think she is. I hear from her now and again). But, her sobriety didn't work very well for me and I broke up with her. I started seeing Denise again and moved back into our house. I finished my Ph.D. and changed jobs again with the goal of trying to get a university faculty position. In this new job, I had the opportunity to attend a week-long seminar on alcohol and drug abuse. The idea was to create intervention teams to help people who had substance abuse problems. This time, I did identify with what the workshop leaders were saying. I was convinced that I was an alcoholic. I actually stopped drinking for about six months. I didn't go to AA or anything. I just stopped.

Why did I start drinking again? Well, I could blame it on a woman but the reality is that I'm an addict and I wasn't doing anything to recover. I started flirting with a woman in my new job and we started fooling around. It wasn't an affair in the technical sense but we were being sexual and romantic and we were both in relationships with others. I told Denise that I wanted to move out (again) but didn't tell her there was another woman. I think I said something about "finding myself" or some other bullshit. The woman I was seeing liked to drink, although I don't think she was alcoholic, and so I joined her. But, once I was really in a relationship with her, I didn't like her so much and broke it off. I stayed in my own place and hid my drinking from Denise. She thought I was still sober.

In the spring of that year, I got a job offer from a university in another state. Denise thought that she and our son would move with me but I told her that I wanted to go alone. From what Denise told me later, she assumed that I would not last long alone and would ask them to come to me after a year or so. But, that never happened.

Now that I was living away from my home town, there was nothing and no one to stop me from doing whatever I wanted to. Nobody knew about my drinking history and I certainly didn't tell anyone. So, I was like a kid in a candy store. I was a single, relatively young professor and I lived a pretty wild life. I got very close to another young professor and his wife and we all liked to smoke dope and drink. So, I was smoking and drinking every day. There was a series of girlfriends and short affairs but nothing serious. I was productive at work and got promoted and tenured at all the normal times. By that time, my tolerance for alcohol was pretty high and I rarely was hung over and I never remember getting out of control. I believe that people thought I was fun. The place where my judgment was probably the most impaired was in the type of women I dated. But, I'm not sure that I can attribute that to my alcohol and drug use.

I do remember becoming aware of how much I drank. When I would come home from work, I would tell myself to just have one or two glasses of wine. But, I would invariably drink the whole bottle. I still had Stoli around and I drank a lot of beer. I don't remember buying a lot of marijuana. Generally, I would help my friends pay for it and would smoke when I was with them. I would go and visit my son about once a month and usually sleep with Denise during these visits. She thought I wasn't drinking so I had to stay sober during these visits. The first thing I did when she would drop me off at the airport was have a drink. One time, Denise and my son visited me. At the time, I was living in a mother-in-law apartment attached to a house. I had done a favor for the owner of the house and he had left a bottle of Stoli for me. I arrived home with Denise and my son and there was the bottle!!! I made up something but I'm sure she was suspicious.

After about six years of this lifestyle, I was tired. I was tired of having a series of relationships, tired of fast food, tired of changing living situations, and tired of being rather decadent. I didn't really focus on having a problem with alcohol and marijuana but I was getting older and thought I should "settle down." My family thought I was a flake and I did too. Still, I was well established professionally and that was my saving grace.

A woman friend introduced me to her girlfriend from high school, who lived about 200 miles away. Let's call her Brenda. She was my age, same religious background, attractive, and a professional in a similar field to mine. We began to date and I was pleased to see that Brenda liked to smoke pot and drink. After about four months of me going back and forth to her house (usually for 2 to 3 days at a time), I proposed. Go ahead and say it. It was stupid but I did it. Brenda wanted me to get a job in her area and move there. But, it was easier for her to get a job in her field than it was for me to get a university job in her area. So, Brenda moved to my town and we moved in together. From the beginning, it was a struggle. Brenda was not happy to move from a job and area she liked. She didn't like her new job. For me, it was a shock to find out that Brenda didn't drink and smoke dope every day. Increasingly, I had to find excuses to drink at night. Before we got married, Brenda told me that she thought I had a drinking problem. I agreed to stop drinking and I did stop for about three years. But, I kept smoking pot. By the time we got married, I knew I was making a mistake but I didn't want my family and friends to have validation that I was a flake so I went through with it. Brenda and I bought a house and she got pregnant. I wanted another kid and figured I could put up with Brenda. Then, she started to get on me about smoking pot. We agreed that smoking about once every couple of months would be OK but I didn't adhere to that very long. But, Brenda was very vigilant and suspicious and she had an amazing sense of smell. So, I had to be very careful. I would take a few tokes before leaving work and would use Visine to get the redness out of my eyes and stop at a gas station and wash my hands and face so I wouldn't smell. I went to great pains to find an isolated spot in my town to smoke. Sometimes, my administrative assistant and a colleague would actually smoke in our office area after everyone had left for the day. We almost got caught once. I would drive home stoned, sometimes in horrendous weather. Sometimes I would smoke while driving. I remember dropping a lit roach in my car one time and I couldn't find it. It is an absolute wonder that I never had an accident or got pulled over. On weekends, Brenda would want to have time away from our child so I would take him and visit friends who smoked. They had a kid too so we would have one of them watch the kids while two of us smoked. Then, the left out person would smoke while the two of us who were already stoned did child duty. I know this is a big rationalization but none of us got out of control so the kids were never in danger. But, of course, I was driving with my kid when I was stoned. A couple of times, Brenda would discover my stash and that would result in a huge confrontation. I would act contrite and agree to go to counseling. But, I never really stopped for any lengthy period of time.

After about six years of marriage, we split up. Brenda was really mad at me but I can't believe it was because she loved me. There hadn't been any sex, affection, or companionship for quite some time. I think she was upset because she hadn't had to work and now she would have to find a job. Financially, I was in bad shape. I was paying child support for my first child, child support and alimony for Brenda and our child, half of the mortgage on our house, and rent for a new place. I didn't make that much money, although it was sufficient for a stable family. I had to borrow money from my parents (I was over 40 at the time) to pay for the divorce attorney. A found a very old, dilapidated house about [a] ½ mile from Brenda's. It was spider-infested and very cold. But, once again, I was on my own and I could do whatever I wanted. Now, I really began to smoke dope on a daily basis. For a few months, I didn't drink but eventually I started drinking again too. I had my child two nights during the week and every other weekend. When we would get home from school, I would put my child in front of the TV and go downstairs and toke up. We did interact but I was always high.

Now, I was absolutely committed to staying single and I really did not want anything to do with women at that point. But, I was horny. I got fixed up with a woman (we'll call her "Kathy") who had been married a couple of times like me and had a child who was about four years older than mine. She was a bit younger than I was but it was less than 10 years so it seemed OK. Now, this is going to be a bit difficult to explain because I need to protect everyone's anonymity. Let's just say that I thought it would be best if she thought I was sober. So, the first time we got together, there was no alcohol or marijuana. Little did I know that she was doing cocaine that night. I didn't have any experience with coke so I would not have known. Anyway, I had some matches on me and she said, "What are those for? Smoking dope?" I was dumbfounded because, given what we both did for a living (which I can't disclose), it was the last thing I expected her to say. But, that opened the door for me.

As much as I resisted getting involved in a relationship, Kathy pushed for one. Eventually, I gave in and I'm glad I did. We are still together today and have a wonderful life. But, that is getting ahead of the story.

Ironically as it may seem, my drug use has increased during the time I have been with Kathy, although my life is more fulfilled than it has ever been. At the beginning of the relationship, there was some marijuana smoking but that was about it. Kathy didn't even really like to smoke and she rarely drank. But, she did introduce me to cocaine. Strangely enough, cocaine never became a big problem for me. We would get some on the weekends and stay out late. I usually drank and smoked dope too. While I did the cocaine compulsively when we had it, I didn't really enjoy it that much. It would keep me awake and fucked up my nose. Kathy didn't seem that wild about it either. Eventually, we stopped getting it and only do it a couple of times a year now. When we do, we usually both say, "Why did we get that shit?" It is usually just on some special occasion or when the guy who gets it for us (he is a regular user and takes a cut when he gets ours) calls to ask if we want some.

About 10 years ago, something happened with Kathy (unrelated to drugs and not something I want to disclose here) that resulted in her wanting to live a more stable life. She wanted me to stop drinking and using drugs and I started going to AA. I have to say that AA is wonderful. The people there are admirable and the philosophy is great. I actually stayed sober for about two years. I think I got bored and complacent and stopped going. Also, the pain pills started.

My major drug problem today involves pain pills, tramadol [the generic name of Ultram] and hydrocodone [generic name of Loratab]. I can't even remember why I started but I think it was some kind of injury. Now Kathy has always loved pain pills and had a doctor who readily prescribed them. But, she never really escalated her use. She would take a steady amount every day. I also found a doctor who never seems to ask many questions about why I need them. So, for the past eight years, I have been taking tramadol every day and hydrocodone occasionally. Just the other day, I told the pharmacist that a relative had been filling my prescription without my knowledge so I could get an early prescription. I have taken pain pills from relatives and friends. Before she died, my mother was living with us. Because of her health issues, she had plenty of pain pills and lots of refills. She didn't like to take them because they made her constipated. But, I took them. Kathy and I volunteered for an elderly woman who was legally blind. I took some of her pain pills. When I go to someone's house, I always go to the bathroom and check out the medicine cabinet. Now, I'm pretty sneaky so I don't take a lot when I find them. So far, I've never been caught as far as I know. When we go to my mother-in-law's, Kathy and I always look through her stash. She has a worse problem than I do. I know that I'm addicted to the pain pills because I've tried to stop a few times and I get withdrawal symptoms. Very unpleasant.

For quite a while, the pain pills were all I was doing. But, a couple of years ago, I started smoking pot and drinking again. The frequency varies. I don't find marijuana that satisfying anymore. It makes me experience self-loathing and I eat too much. I like alcohol but Kathy doesn't really like me to drink and it's too hard to hide. So, I sneak a beer now and then but the only time I really drink a lot is when Kathy is out of town or I go out of town. Even with that, I have found that I don't really have the desire to overdo it. The last time Kathy was out of town, I bought a bottle of Stoli and threw most of it away. I guess age is catching up with me. So, I know that today is a little unusual. On most days, it is just the pills, usually four to eight, depending on what I have. I might smoke a little on the weekend.

I guess that is the whole drug story. Like I said, I'm not proud of what I am doing and want to stop. But, I do have to say that my life is as good as it has ever been. Kathy and I make a good living and we really enjoy each other's company. We have great relationships with our children. I do community volunteer work and am active in other areas. Now, if I can just stop taking those damn pills. . . .

Analysis of Mark

Of the three functional addicts described in this chapter, Mark has the most serious problem with alcohol and other drugs. He could probably be diagnosed with a substance dependence disorder. Reviewing the criteria to diagnose this condition in Chapter 1, you will recall that at least three of the seven criteria must be present in any 12-month period. There is evidence that Mark meets the first five criteria. Mark has described symptoms of both tolerance and withdrawal, the first two criteria. Remember, tolerance means that an increasing amount of the substance is needed to produce the desired effect. While Mark alludes to this when describing how many pills he takes, I do know from other information (again, I cannot divulge anything about this) that Mark has to take many more pills than the recommended dose to experience any euphoria. He does say that he has experienced withdrawal symptoms when he has attempted to discontinue his use of pills. The third criterion involves taking a larger amount of alcohol or other drugs or over a longer period of time than intended. Mark's story contains many references to this. This criterion may be a little "iffy," since it is difficult to determine if it has occurred recently. From Mark's story, it sounds like his alcohol and marijuana use is fairly controlled at this point. However, he has said in other contacts that if he has access to pills, he uses more than he intends to. Mark generally limits his access to pills by having his partner hide them. The fourth criterion is a persistent desire or unsuccessful efforts to control the use of alcohol and other drugs. Mark clearly indicates that he wants to discontinue this use and relates times he has tried to quit. Finally, the fifth criterion includes spending a great deal of time making sure that substances are available. Mark describes many examples of this, particularly with regard to pills. In fact, Mark and his partner have made hiding pills a game between them. Mark's partner takes pride in finding good places to hide the pills and Mark spends a lot of time looking for them.

If Mark can be diagnosed with a substance dependence disorder, how can he be a functional addict? In other words, it seems to make some inherent sense that those who are diagnosed with the least severe substance use disorder (substance abuse) may be able to function adequately but those with a substance dependence disorder should not be able to proceed in life undetected. There are several different explanations. The first involves the diagnostic criteria for the two conditions. There has been some discussion in the professional literature regarding the accuracy of the distinction between substance abuse disorders and substance dependence disorders. Although this book is not about these kinds of issues, some explanation is necessary to clarify Mark's inclusion as a functional addict.

It is clear when examining the diagnostic criteria for the two conditions that the criteria for substance abuse disorders involves "trouble" resulting from alcohol and other drug use. In contrast, the diagnostic criteria for substance dependence disorders are almost all related to the substance itself as opposed to the consequences of alcohol and other drug use. Therefore, although Mark does meet the criteria for a substance dependence disorder, it doesn't logically follow that his condition is more serious than someone who has been arrested for a DUI. However, according to the DSM-IV TR, Mark cannot be diagnosed with a substance abuse disorder for any category of drugs when he meets the definition of a substance dependence disorder for that class of drugs. With regard to pain pills (opioid drugs), Mark can be diagnosed with an opioid dependence disorder. At this point, he probably does not meet the criteria for an alcohol abuse disorder or a cannabis (marijuana) abuse disorder. So, while he technically can be diagnosed with the more serious substance dependence disorder, it is not clear that he has had more problems from his alcohol and other drug use than someone who has been diagnosed with the less serious substance abuse disorder. Parenthetically, the DSM-IV TR is being revised and the distinctions between the two substance use disorders will hopefully be clarified.

Another explanation for Mark's continuing "success" in remaining an undetected addict has to do with something discussed at the beginning of this chapter. Although I can't find any research to substantiate this clinical observation, a persistent distinction I have found between functional addicts and disease model addicts involves the effects of alcohol and other drugs on behavior. It is very common to hear stories from disease model addicts about the very significant behavior changes they experienced when under the influence of alcohol and other drugs. Although the behavior changes are not the same from one person to the next, they are always dramatic. Some people become violent, some extroverted, some obnoxious, some morose. Disease model addicts will tell stories about doing things they never would have thought themselves capable of when sober.

Functional addicts do not report these kinds of significant behavior change when under the influence. You may recall in George's story that he talked about always wanting to be in control of his behavior and that one thing he disliked about LSD was that he did not always feel in control. In Mark's long history of alcohol and other drug use, he only described one blackout and he says that his behavior didn't change much when he was intoxicated. Perhaps there are physiological differences between functional addicts and disease model addicts that account for these behavioral differences. Mark's reaction to cocaine certainly suggests that his physiology is different than many other addicts. Cocaine is a highly addictive substance and many people have had significant problems related to its use. Mark says that cocaine never had much effect on him even though he used it compulsively when it was available.

Finally, it is clear that Mark has been lucky. When he drove while intoxicated, he never had an accident or was ever pulled over by the police. He smoked marijuana in his car during inclement weather at night on a dangerous freeway. While some of this "luck" may be attributed to the relative lack of significant behavior change while intoxicated, he had no control over other drivers. Mark could have easily been involved in an accident and his drug use detected as part of the routine investigation. That would have significantly changed his circumstances.

Interview with Amy

Amy is a 52-year-old woman who is a very successful business executive. She is married to her third husband, who she has been with for 13 years. She has one adult daughter who she is very close to. Amy is a recovering compulsive gambler who has remained abstinent for over 12 years.

I: What was your first experience with alcohol and other drugs?

A: Do you want me to start with cigarettes?

I: Sure.

A: I remember when I was 12. I remember stealing one of my mother's cigarettes and trying it. I was 12. Alcohol, I have to think about one. I guess I was 12 and my mom was out of town. I had some friends over and we got into the alcohol. I remember marijuana. I was 16 or just turning 16. Yeah, I was probably 15 and I went to a concert with some older people and they were smoking pot and I tried it then.

I: Did you get high?

A: No, I don't remember the first time I got high. I do know that in high school after that experience, I would smoke hash in my room. I would put it under glass. You take a little bit of hash because it's a chunk, and put it on a safety pin. You put it under a glass and light it kind of like incense. Then you move the glass to the end of the counter or something and inhale it. I did that a lot in my room because it didn't smell.

I: By yourself?

A: Yeah, I did it a lot by myself but I did it with my friends too. So I was probably around 15 when I started. I think I tried acid once during that timeframe. I was living in [name of state] with my mom. But, Quaaludes were big. Did a lot of Quaaludes.

I: How old?

A: I really got into Quaaludes when I moved to [name of city] when I was about 17, 18, 19. I did a lot of those. I never really abused drugs. I guess as a young adult when I was with [name of first husband] I drank a lot. But it wasn't like a daily thing. You know, the lifestyle in [name of city] was going to a bar. That's when I learned to gamble. They had started to put the machines in and I didn't know what they were. I got interested. Now all of a sudden I had something to do when I was at the bars. I was mesmerized. But as far as drugs and alcohol and marijuana, I don't want to make it sound like I didn't do it a lot but I don't know. I really can't remember. I don't think it was a really big deal. I probably smoked a lot of pot. When I was . . . I do remember that. So, I smoked a lot of marijuana in high school and in college I smoked a lot.

I: What's that mean? Every day?

A: Yeah, OK. So now I'm in [city where she went to college]. Let's fast forward. This I remember. I was 19. And, I would drive home a lot. Like one time I had a boyfriend here. From [name of city] to [name of city]. I would smoke the whole way. I had a little . . . I was really into Ziggie, that character? I had a little box with Ziggie on it and I had all my paraphernalia in there and I would smoke all the way from [name of city] to here and back. But, drinking. I drank. I don't know. I never really think about this, so. . . . Marijuana was more my thing in high school and college and pills, Quaaludes. We were really into those. So I did a lot of those. I remember I burned my leg on a motorcycle and I didn't feel it. I was high and I was on Quaaludes. I almost needed medical attention. I was riding on the back on a guy's motorcycle and I didn't feel it. My leg was against the exhaust and didn't feel it.

I: So, what happened?

A: Well, when I realized it we put some ointment on it. I just hurt like hell for a while. But, at that point in time, it didn't hurt me. I must have been pretty wasted, huh?

I: Did you have any other consequences as a result of alcohol and other drugs?

A: I don't ever remember wrecking my car

I: Did you ever get busted?

A: By my mother, never had an incident with the police.

I: Sexual assault or anything?

A: Well, I slept with a lot of boys. I was pretty promiscuous. I was aware of what I was doing but I was making very bad decisions. I was very reckless. Today I can see that I wanted attention. I wanted to be accepted and loved. If I had sex with a boy, I thought that was what that meant. So I was pretty sexually active. And when I was sexually active, I would either be high or on Quaaludes. I'm trying to think of when I started to do cocaine.

Umm, I don't remember the first time I did it. But, when I was with [name of second husband], because [name of second husband] had a cocaine problem, I did a lot of cocaine. A lot of coke.

I: How old were you?

A: Well, I had [name of daughter] when I was 27. So, 28, 29, 30, 31. Well, I also freebased cocaine occasionally with [name of first husband] but that wasn't frequent.

I: When you say a lot of cocaine, what do you mean? Every day?

A: [name of second husband] did it every day. I don't remember me doing it every day but I remember a lot. Like several times a week at least. Definitely on the weekends. I guess we did it during the week too. Then I introduced him to gambling. He never gambled before. And, it was horrible. So, on the nights when [name of daughter] was with [name of first husband], we'd be gambling and doing cocaine. And, then regulate it with Adivan. Then [name of friend] and I did it but not often. I ripped her off sometimes. One time I put sweet and low in it. She was pissed. She thought [name of drug dealer] did it. I remember when I got into pain pills. I remember exactly when I got in to those. My mom broke her ankle. So, I was always into scamming pills whenever anyone had them but I remember going over there and stealing them when she wasn't home. [name of housekeeper] would give them to me. So, I've been doing pain pills since whenever she broke her foot which is at least 12 years.

I: How do you get them?

A: Prescriptions. Well, I pushed the envelope to get the prescriptions. I used to get them from my OB/GYN. Then he moved so I had to start hustling them. I remember when I got the biggest batch of Loratabs that was from Dr. [name of doctor], he wrote a prescription of 120. I thought, "What the fuck?" Who does that? One time, we were on vacation in southern California and we went to Mexico and bought a lot of different pills. That kept us going for a while.

I: Have you ever had to get them illegally?

A: One time I got some illegal pills from one of my daughter's girlfriends before we went on vacation one summer. She was able to get oxycodone and a lot of other ones too. This is really terrible but there was this close friend of a friend who was dying of cancer. After she died, I volunteered to gather up her unused prescriptions and "donate" them. But, I took all the pain meds and kept them. There was a lot of them too and some really good stuff. But, usually I didn't have to do that kind of stuff because I have always known doctors. [name of doctor friend] used to write them for me. I forgot about that. So, before I got them from the OB guy, [name of doctor friend] used to write me prescriptions. Now, I'm about to run out. I only have one prescription left.

I: So, today, how many pills do you take a day?

A: During the week? I try not to take any more than two or three. But, it has probably been more like three lately because I've developed such a tolerance. Today, I've probably taken four. 'Cause, I don't feel them anymore. It's a drag. I don't feel them at all. Once in a while, I get a little buzz. So, it's kind of worthless. I need to get off of them.

Analysis of Amy

Amy was very reluctant to participate in the interview. She resisted going into depth about her drug use. I suspect that she was minimizing the extent of her pill use but I do not have any firm evidence to substantiate that suspicion. It was also difficult to get her to go into detail about incidents from her past, so there may have been many more examples about consequences from alcohol and other drug use than she was willing to admit. However, I do know that she did not omit any serious consequences that have occurred in her recent past. Again, I can't be more specific than that but "recent past" includes multiple years.

With regard to diagnosis, her situation is similar to that of Mark. Technically, she could be diagnosed with a substance dependence disorder. Amy did describe tolerance to pain pills (e.g., "I don't feel them anymore"), a desire to quit (e.g., "I need to get off of them."), and spending a lot of time in her efforts to ensure a supply of pain pills, as evidenced by her description of going to different doctors. Therefore, Amy has demonstrated three of the criteria necessary for a diagnosis of a substance dependence disorder. I would suspect she would have withdrawal symptoms if she tried to discontinue her use but she did not discuss this and I have no knowledge of any previous efforts to stop.

As with Mark, it would be difficult to diagnose Amy with a substance abuse disorder because she did not really describe any serious consequences as a result of her alcohol and other drug use and there have not been any consequences in the past 12 months (the necessary time period to diagnose a substance abuse disorder). Similar to Mark, this may say something about the validity of the diagnostic categories of substance abuse disorders and substance dependence disorders, particularly in regard to the concept that substance dependence disorders are more serious than substance abuse disorders.

In the introduction to Amy, I said that she was a recovering compulsive gambler with 12 years of abstinence. Amy does not mention her gambling in her interview, except when she says that she introduced her cocaine-abusing second husband to gambling. While gambling addiction is not the topic of this book, it adds a dimension to Amy's case that is relevant in that it contradicts conventional thinking about addiction. As was the case with George and Mark, I can't divulge how I know this information about Amy's gambling problem but I know it was extremely serious and easily met the criteria for Pathological Gambling in the DSM-IV TR. She sought help for her gambling addiction and attended Gamblers Anonymous (GA) for about the first five years of her recovery. Although she no longer attends GA meetings, Amy has remained abstinent from gambling.

The traditional view of addiction is that those individuals who develop problems with one type of addictive activity (alcohol and other drugs, gambling, shopping) are prone to develop addiction with other activities. In other words, most treatment providers would predict that Amy would have the same problems with alcohol and other drugs as she has with gambling. There is some research evidence to support this. A well-known epidemiological study of alcoholism and related conditions published in 2005 found that nearly three quarters of pathological gamblers had an alcohol use disorder and over 38% had another drug use disorder.[1]

The question is "How can Amy have a serious pathological gambling disorder and be able to maintain a functional-use pattern with regard to alcohol and other drugs?" Although there is no way to definitively answer this question since there is so little research on functional addicts, Amy seems to share characteristics with George and Mark in that she does not seem to experience any major behavioral changes when she is under the influence of alcohol and other drugs and she does not lose her ability to maintain some control over her drug use. When Amy says that she doesn't feel much of an effect from pain pills, she does not report increasing the number of pills she takes. As any treatment provider can attest, individuals with pain pill dependence report increasing their intake as tolerance develops. In many cases, they will be taking enough pills to kill a nontolerant person. Now, tramadol (the generic name for Ultram and one of the types of pain pills Amy takes) is not an opioid, although it is addictive. Perhaps it is the type of pill Amy takes that accounts for her "control." However, Amy did not discuss her use of hydrocodone (generic name of Loratab), which is an opioid (as with all the information I add to the interviews and stories, I cannot say how I know this). She does get prescriptions of hydrocodone, but her use pattern is very similar to her use of tramadol. When she has hydrocodone, she uses it daily and has developed a tolerance to it. However, she does not increase her dose.

CONCLUSION

Until functional addicts become the focus of research efforts, much of what we can conclude about the largest subtype of addicts is conjecture based on these three cases and my own and others' clinical and personal experiences. It may be surprising that there hasn't been research on this type of addict, since some of the suspicions about the differences between functional addicts and disease model addicts have important implications for treatment. However, there would be practical barriers to studying this population, the most obvious being a realistic method to identify and thoroughly interview functional addicts. If you recall, the population from the original study that identified subtypes of alcoholics was derived from a large sample in the National Epidemiological Survey on Alcohol and Related Conditions (described in Chapter 1). Prior to the data analysis, the researchers did not know what subtypes they would identify. Now, the investigators did conduct personal interviews with each subject and it might be possible, depending on how the data were coded, to re-interview the subjects and test some of the hypothetical differences between functional and disease addicts. This would be an expensive and time-consuming process and the sample was limited to alcohol dependence rather than any other drug dependence so there would be problems generalizing the results to all addicts. None of our functional case studies involved significant alcohol use. However, a very skilled and ambitious young researcher could create a very productive academic career if he or she could secure grant funding to study this group. I am too close to retirement to go down this road.

With the disease model addicts and ASPD addicts, it is easier to get access to research populations. Disease model addicts are found in treatment facilities and ASPD addicts are found either in treatment or in correctional settings. Identifying functional addicts probably would entail recruitment from the general population (e.g., an advertisement on Craigslist). This type of self-selection would likely produce a biased sample. As I noted earlier, I found functional addicts who were not willing to tell me their stories and I would suspect that many functional addicts would not be motivated to self-identify to a researcher they knew nothing about.

Therefore, we are left with drawing conclusions from a very small sample that is unlikely to be representative of the population of functional addicts. After all, are three had professional positions and two had advanced college degrees. However, there still are some intriguing similarities in the three case examples. First, all three of our functional addicts have been extremely fortunate to have avoided any accidents or serious encounters with law enforcement. As we saw with George, he was pulled over once in a situation that could have resulted in a lot of problems for him. However, although it's hard to deny that there is an element of luck in the cases of the functional addicts, they also tend to avoid many high-risk situations and their relatively inconspicuous behavior changes when under the influence do not draw attention to them. So, luck is also related to the other factors that seem to differentiate functional addicts from disease model addicts.

These other factors and the relationship between them seem to be the elements that require research attention. That is, the functional addicts we have described all have a high tolerance for alcohol and other drugs, do not show significant behavior changes when under the influence, and exercise more control than disease model addicts in regard to when, where, and how much alcohol and other drugs they use.

In the last few years, there has been increasing research attention to and funding at the federal level for the neurobiology of addiction, with the National Institute on Drug Abuse the lead federal agency in this effort. A logical hypothesis to test would be that there are neurobiological differences between disease model addicts and functional addicts. If evidence can be found to support this hypothesis, it would have significant implications in the treatment of addicts. These implications are discussed in the next chapter.

FIVE

Implications for Intervention and Treatment

INTRODUCTION

Up to this point, this book has been a description of subtypes of addicts. Although I hope you have found this discussion interesting, you would be justified in saying "So what?" Simply knowing that there are subtypes does not solve the problems of getting addicts into treatment and increasing the number of addicts who complete treatment. This chapter addresses those problems.

Before proceeding, I need to dampen expectations. It is unrealistic to think that many or even most of the 22 million Americans with a substance use disorder will "see the light" and seek treatment. Even if they did, there is not sufficient capacity in the treatment system to deal with them. But, the main reason why not all of the people who need treatment are going to seek it has to do with the nature of these disorders. To understand this, think about a lifestyle problem such as obesity. People know they are overweight and they know it is better if they are not overweight. But, most obese people do not lose weight. They may start a diet and exercise program and give up or they just may never try. It is just the nature of human behavior. Lifestyle changes are difficult, they are not fun, and the status quo usually has a pleasurable component. Along with that, alcohol and other drug problems are stigmatized for many Americans. So, for many people with substance use disorders, admitting to a problem with alcohol or other drugs is admitting to a personal weakness. For these reasons, there will probably always be a very sizeable number of people with substance use disorders who do not get help.

PUBLIC HEALTH POLICY

There have been a couple of examples of public health issues involving lifestyle change where intense public awareness campaigns combined with public policy changes have resulted in significant behavioral modifications in a large proportion of the population. Wearing seat belts in cars is one example. When I was young, there were no seat belts in cars. Even when cars were mandated to include seat belts, we never wore them. After many years, intense public awareness campaigns, and fines for not wearing seat belts, most people now routinely wear them. However, you still hear about accidents where serious injuries occurred because passengers were not wearing seat belts.

A public health issue that is closely related to alcohol and drug problems is cigarette smoking. When I started college in 1969, we were allowed to smoke in class. A pack of cigarettes cost 35 cents and there plenty of vending machines dispensing cigarettes. The Surgeon General's report on the health dangers of smoking had already been issued, so knowledge about the relationship between cigarettes and serious illness was already out there. After many years of public awareness efforts, increases in tobacco taxes, and restrictions on marketing, distribution, and places that allow smoking, there has been a significant decrease in the number of people who smoke. However, nearly 24% of people still smoke.[1]

Therefore, it would theoretically be possible to reduce the number of people who drink and use illicit drugs through a combination of intense public awareness, restrictions on access, aggressive law enforcement, and increased excise taxes (for alcohol). During prohibition, there was a significant reduction in alcohol consumption and in the problems resulting from alcohol abuse. However, there is no public appetite for this kind of effort because of the inconvenience it causes for those who use alcohol moderately and because of the amount of law enforcement resources required to enforce restrictions on alcohol. Furthermore, such efforts are more effective at limiting the use of those who rarely have problems anyway. Most people with substance use disorders are motivated to get their source of alcohol and other drugs regardless of the barriers. However, there would probably be preventative value in an intense combination of public awareness and public policy changes regarding alcohol and illicit drugs. In other words, such efforts might discourage some of those who have the potential to develop problems from using alcohol and illicit drugs.

Because there is no political will to aggressively attack alcohol and illicit drug use from a public health perspective, this is largely an academic discussion. Furthermore, I am not advocating such an approach. It is not clear that the cost of the resources necessary to conduct a campaign similar to that which was done with cigarettes would be worth it. However, there is evidence that pubic policies with regard to alcohol can impact alcohol use and the negative consequences associated with alcohol abuse. This is particularly true in regard to underage drinking.[2] Therefore, increases in excise taxes, restrictions on retail outlets, sting operations, server training, "use it and lose it" laws (i.e., underage drinkers lose their driver's license), and other public policies should be more broadly implemented.

RECOMMENDATIONS FOR ALL SUBTYPES

Regardless of subtype, there are some things that can be done to improve treatment access, retention, and effectiveness. Although these recommendations are not specific to any one subtype, they are a result of the total information regarding subtypes.

Treatment of co-occurring disorders: For some time, federal officials, researchers, and treatment providers have known that a high percentage of individuals with a substance use disorder have a co-occurring mental disorder. According to the Center for Substance Abuse Treatment, over half of those with lifetime alcohol abuse or alcohol dependence disorder also had a serious mental illness in their lifetime. This figure rose to nearly 60% for those with an illicit drug abuse or dependence disorder and was over 70% for people with alcohol and illicit drug disorders.[3] The most common types of these mental disorders include mood disorders (e.g., major depressive disorder, dysthymic disorder, bipolar disorder), anxiety disorders (e.g., panic disorders, phobias, obsessive-compulsive disorder, posttraumatic stress disorder, generalized anxiety disorder), and personality disorders. We have already thoroughly discussed antisocial personality disorder but there are other personality disorders as well. Occasionally, a psychotic disorder such as schizophrenia may occur.

In the description of the subtypes in Chapter 1, the Intermediate Familial, Young Antisocial, and Chronic Severe subtypes had the highest proportion of people with co-occurring mental disorders. Since these subtypes were also the most likely to have been in treatment, it is not surprising that such a high proportion of clients in treatment for a substance use disorder have a co-occurring mental disorder.

Although it would seem to make sense to treat both the substance use disorder and the co-occurring mental disorder simultaneously, this has not always been the case. A common school of thought in substance abuse treatment was that the substance use disorder should be treated first and other mental disorders treated after stable recovery had been established. An example demonstrates why this usually doesn't work. Imagine a 32-year-old woman in treatment for a methamphetamine addiction. She reports a history of childhood sexual abuse from her step-father and, as a result, suffers from post-traumatic stress disorder (PTSD). The client responds well to substance abuse treatment and remains abstinent for four weeks. Prior to treatment, this woman had been numbing herself against the intense, negative emotions from her history of sexual abuse. Now that she is no longer using drugs, the emotions flood back. If the treatment providers are not attending to the PTSD, she won't be able to cope with these feelings and she relapses.

This problem would seem to have a straightforward solution: treat the substance use disorder and the co-occurring mental disorder simultaneously. Unfortunately, in many states, the substance abuse treatment systems and the mental health treatment systems are separate. Often, substance abuse treatment providers do not have the training and certification or licensure required to treat other mental disorders. Conversely, many mental health treatment providers are not adequately trained in substance use disorders. Even when substance abuse treatment programs have the desire to offer co-occurring disorder treatment services, they may not have the financial resources to hire mental health providers such as psychiatrists, psychologists, mental health counselors, and social workers. Very often, the treatment of co-occurring disorders requires medications that can only be prescribed and managed by a psychiatrist and that is expensive.

While there has been progress in this area in the last 10 years, it is essential that the substance abuse treatment and mental health treatment systems be fully integrated and that more treatment providers gain the training and certification or licensure to treat both substance use disorders and other mental disorders.

Recovery Oriented Systems of Care: Regardless of what subtype we are talking about, it is clear that substance use disorders are chronic conditions that cannot be "cured" and which do not usually go into remission following an episode of acute care. In other words, most people who go to treatment and do not do some kind of structured follow-up for a very long time (or the rest of their lives) relapse. One reason Alcoholics Anonymous is so popular and works so well for those who regularly attend is that the meetings provide regular, consistent, and structured follow-up and support. By saying this, I am not trying to disparage or to dispute the concept that the spiritual aspect of Twelve Step recovery groups is the essential ingredient for success. Apart from whether this is true or not, there is no disagreement among professionals that regular attendance at meetings keeps a recovering individual focused on sobriety, provides social support from others who have similar experiences, and offers a structure for how to progress in recovery. With any chronic condition, regular follow-up is important. I have high cholesterol and high blood sugar, and my physician encourages me to schedule regular follow-up appointments to monitor my blood and my weight. We discuss lifestyle management and he makes suggestions in areas I am struggling with. Recovery from a substance use disorder requires the same (or greater) level of contact with a professional or peers who offer feedback and support.

Again, there seems to be an obvious and simple solution: encourage recovering individuals to attend AA or NA. And, that works very well for many people. However, not everyone is comfortable with Twelve Step meetings, and many recovering individuals have multiple needs that cannot be met through support group meetings alone. The term "Recovery Oriented Systems of Care" has been used to describe the range of services including screening, assessment, detoxification, acute treatment, and recovery management. Recovery management can include follow-up visits with mental health professionals or family counseling; support group attendance; financial, legal, vocational, and/or educational guidance; and peer recovery-support services. Peer recovery-support services involves recovering individuals who provide information, advice, and support to other recovering individuals. For example, ex-offenders who are recovering can be extremely helpful to recovering individuals who are transitioning from an institution. There are also peer recovery-support groups for the LGBT (lesbian, gay, bisexual, and transgender) community, women, and specific ethnic groups.

Harm Management: In Chapter 1, it was noted that less than 10% of the people who need treatment for a substance use disorder actually received treatment. While the goal of getting more of these folks into treatment is admirable, it is also realistic to acknowledge that the vast majority of people who need treatment are not going to get it. However, many of these people who do not get treatment will cause problems for themselves, their friends and family, their employers, and for society. The list of these problems is very long but can include traffic accidents, domestic violence, crimes committed to get money for alcohol and other drugs, reduced productivity at work, family disruption, emergency room visits, emotional distress for loved ones, and so on. It seems prudent to take steps to reduce the harm caused by those who have untreated substance use disorders.

There are some harm-management (usually called "harm-reduction") measures that are already widely accepted in this country. For example, methadone maintenance for opioid addicts is a very effective harm-management technique. Rather than using heroin, the addict is administered a substitute opioid, methadone, through a registered clinic. The person is still addicted to opioids but is able to function and does not have to engage in illegal activity to get and use heroin.

There are other harm-management procedures that are used in local communities but that are not sanctioned by the federal government. The most common of these is needle-exchange programs. Addicts who inject drugs can exchange a used needle for a clean one. These programs have been shown to reduce the spread of diseases such as HIV and hepatitis. Until recently, the federal government has banned the use of federal funds to support needle-exchange programs. The Obama Administration supports ending this restriction.

Other harm-management programs are used in other countries but not in the United States. There are heroin distribution programs where heroin is provided for registered addicts, drug-checking programs that assess the safety of drugs like ecstasy at rave parties, and drug-consumption rooms where registered addicts can inject drugs in a safe, supervised setting. Obviously, these harm-management programs are controversial and there does not seem to be the political will to experiment with them in this country. Since the alternative seems to be to do nothing and to continue to have the serious consequences of alcohol and other drug abuse, it would certainly seem to be worthwhile to consider the implementation of more harm-management programs in this country.

Treatment Providers: For those who are interested in the history of addiction treatment, the seminal work in this area is a book by William White, an advocate for the recovery community, titled *Slaying the Dragon: The History of Addiction Treatment and Recovery in America.*[4] Providers of addiction treatment services in the first formal treatment programs in the mid-1900s were recovering alcoholics (these initial programs were only for alcoholics). There were no academic training programs for addiction-treatment providers. As treatment programs spread across the country, states adopted certification requirements for alcohol and drug counselors but these standards were oriented towards the counselor who was a recovering addict. For example, the only formal education required was a high school diploma or GED. In the early 1990s, the federal government instituted grant programs to encourage colleges and universities to implement formal training programs for addiction-treatment providers and for states to increase the certification standards for addiction counselors. Although these efforts have dramatically improved the training of addiction treatment providers, most states still have initial certification for addiction counselors at the bachelor's level. This means that addiction counselors have less formal training than other behavioral health care providers such as clinical social workers, marriage and family therapists, and mental health counselors, who all must have at least a master's degree.

The evolution of the profession of addiction counseling has been impacted by two competing forces. The field of addiction treatment has become increasingly complex due to the diversity of the patient population in terms of gender, ethnicity, age, sexual orientation, and drugs of choice. Furthermore, as we have already discussed, many or most patients in addiction treatment have co-occurring mental disorders and many have significant legal, health, and financial problems. Obviously, providing treatment services for this population requires well-trained professional staff. On the other hand, the addiction-treatment field has a long-standing tradition of utilizing recovering individuals as addiction counselors. There has always been resistance to imposing requirements that hinder the ability of recovering individuals without formal academic training to enter the field.

While there is no simple way to resolve these competing forces, many formal training programs in colleges and universities have aggressively recruited and mentored recovering individuals who want to become addiction counselors. As someone who has been involved in these efforts for the last 17 years, I have found the combination of recovery status and formal training to be very powerful. Our recovering students who have earned master's degrees have become program directors and have become involved in state and national addiction treatment initiatives.

An additional issue that impacts the quality of addiction treatment providers is salary. The salary for these providers has historically been very low, even by the standards for behavioral health care providers who traditionally do not make large salaries. The poor pay has been related to the fact that addiction counselors typically did not have advanced degrees but also to the recovery status of most treatment providers. The idea of a recovering person becoming an addiction counselor was viewed as a "mission" as opposed to a career. In other words, many recovering individuals perceived the concept of helping other addicts in treatment settings as their way of repaying the help they had received. This would be consistent with the 12th step of Alcoholics Anonymous ("Having had a spiritual awakening as the result of these steps, we tried to carry this message to alcoholics, and to practice these principles in all our affairs") and a focus on service in Twelve Step groups. Therefore, money was not the primary motivating force for a recovering person to become a treatment provider and, in fact, the low salary contributed to a sense of mission among addiction counselors. In addition, many addiction counselors work in public sector treatment programs, where money is usually sparse.

In order for addiction treatment to become more effective, treatment providers must be adequately trained in the use of evidence-based practices and must be able to work with the diverse treatment population they will encounter. Because of the high proportion of patients with substance use disorders and co-occurring mental disorders, addiction treatment providers should be able to diagnose and treat (with consultation from other professionals) some co-occurring mental disorders. However, if entry into the profession requires more training, the salary for addiction counseling must be commensurate with other behavioral health care providers. In order to ensure that recovering individuals continue to be part of the provider network, active outreach and mentoring to the recovery community must be undertaken.

TREATMENT INTERVENTIONS FOR DISEASE MODEL ADDICTS

The traditional treatment system works fairly well for disease model addicts, assuming they do not have a co-occurring mental disorder. Obviously, the ideas mentioned in the previous section in regard to the treatment of co-occurring disorders and recovery oriented systems of care would increase the effectiveness of treatment for disease model addicts.

Traditional treatment has been based on the idea that all addicts fit the disease model. The treatment approach is called the Minnesota Model, developed by the Hazeldon Foundation in the 1940s and 1950s and based on the principles of Alcoholics Anonymous. A continuum of care including assessment and diagnosis, detoxification, inpatient services, therapeutic communities, halfway houses, outpatient services, and aftercare has been developed using the Minnesota Model. Most people are familiar with the Betty Ford Center in California (a Minnesota Model treatment program), where many famous people have gone for inpatient treatment. In the Minnesota Model, group therapy is used and is concerned with present and future behavior as opposed to past causal factors. Groups are often confrontational. The family also receives therapy. Didactic experiences, including lectures and videotapes, are used to educate clients about the disease of addiction and the consequences of the disease. Although the staff is composed of professionals from a number of disciplines (physicians, social workers, psychologists, nurses, and clergy), recovering addicts and alcoholics are also used as counselors. Clients have reading and writing assignments, such as reading the AA Twelve Steps and Twelve Traditions and writing their life histories. Attendance at AA/NA meetings is required, and clients are expected to work through the first three to five steps of AA while in treatment. There may also be work assignments and recreational activities, depending on the treatment setting. Aftercare includes attendance at AA or NA meetings. Obviously, abstinence from all mind-altering substances is the treatment goal. There is certainly nothing wrong with this approach to treating disease model addicts. And, to be fair, many programs that are based on the Minnesota Model have incorporated evidence-based practices to improve treatment outcomes. For example, the concept of using harsh confrontation in group therapy has largely been discredited and replaced with strategies from an approach called "motivational interviewing" (a series of counseling strategies based on a client's readiness to change). Most of the problems with the traditional approach to treatment have been that is not effective with addicts who do not fit the disease model, it is insufficient in working with addicts with co-occurring mental disorders, and it lacks the long-term recovery management that is necessary to sustain lifestyle changes.

Since the Minnesota Model is based on the principles of Alcoholics Anonymous, it is reasonable to question the necessity of high-cost treatment when AA is free and widely available. It is also true that many severe addicts have achieved long-term, stable recovery through regular attendance at Twelve Step meetings and never going through formal treatment (e.g., the case example of Steve in Chapter 2). The problem is predicting who will be the most likely to achieve recovery through attendance at Twelve Step meetings alone. We know that disease model addicts with co-occurring mental disorders probably need treatment in addition to whatever interventions are used for the substance use disorder. Of course, attendance at Twelve Step meetings does not preclude a person from seeking help for other problems. However, as was noted in the first section of this chapter, treatment for substance use disorders and treatment for co-occurring mental disorders should be fully integrated and this would not be the case if a person was relying solely on Twelve Step meetings for recovery from a substance use disorder. Therefore, for disease model addicts with co-occurring disorders, formal treatment is warranted in most cases, and we can only hope that treatment for substance use disorders and treatment for other mental disorders become more fully integrated.

The detoxification process is another issue that must be considered in determining how to proceed with a disease model addict. For central nervous system depressants such as alcohol or minor tranquilizers, the detoxification process can be medically dangerous and, therefore, should occur in a supervised environment for those with central nervous system-depressant dependence and/or those with serious medical conditions. For central nervous system stimulants (e.g., cocaine, methamphetamine) or opioids (e.g., heroin, oxycodone), withdrawal can be extremely unpleasant but is not generally dangerous from a medical standpoint. People can and do go "cold turkey" without formal detoxification. However, a lot of people also relapse during the withdrawal process because it is so uncomfortable. So, people who are dependent on central nervous system stimulants or opioids and who are otherwise healthy can either detoxify in a supervised setting or on their own. But, if someone has tried unsuccessfully to detoxify on his or her own, a supervised setting is recommended.

For a lot of disease model addicts, the recovery process has many starts and stops before stable recovery is achieved (if it is ever achieved). An addict may start with Twelve Step meetings, relapse, go to formal treatment, relapse, go back to meetings and achieve stable recovery. There are many permutations of this sequence and they can include other interventions such as private therapy, acupuncture, physicians, religious institutions, and others strategies (e.g., the example of Melinda in Chapter 2). So, the bottom line regarding treatment for disease model addicts is that traditional treatment, Twelve Step support groups, a combination of the two, or other alternative interventions may be effective. It is not possible to predict which type of approach or which combination of approaches will work and, frequently, multiple episodes of interventions will occur before stable recovery is achieved. Unfortunately, in too many cases, recovery does not occur.

TREATMENT INTERVENTIONS FOR ANTISOCIAL PERSONALITY DISORDER (ASPD) ADDICTS

In Chapter 3, APSD was discussed thoroughly. It was pointed out that ASPD addicts should be treated separately from disease model addicts. So, there is a necessity for a comprehensive assessment at the beginning of the treatment process and this assessment must include professionals with the training and licensure to diagnose personality disorders. In most states, this involves a psychologist or a psychiatrist. However, in far too many situations, a comprehensive assessment is not conducted nor do psychologists and psychiatrists participate in the assessment process. Furthermore, the diagnosis of personality disorders (or other mental disorders for that matter) is not a precise science. Different professionals from the same discipline can reach different diagnostic decisions.

Many, if not most, ASPD addicts are treated within the criminal justice system in jails, prisons, or therapeutic communities. Therefore, they are often fairly well segregated. Of course, there are still a lot of disease model addicts who become involved in the criminal justice system and ASPD addicts who are diverted from incarceration through drug courts or who avoid arrest. The point is that because of imprecise diagnosis and the fact that disease model addicts and ASPD addicts may end up in the same treatment setting, it may not be possible to keep disease model addicts and ASPD addicts separated in the treatment process. However, this is the desired outcome. If it is not possible to achieve this outcome prior to the beginning of the treatment process, it may be possible shortly after the treatment process begins, because ASPD addicts will often be the most resistive and acting-out clients.

The case example of Henry in Chapter 3 showed that some success with ASPD clients is possible. Now, his story is told from his perspective and so he did portray himself more favorably than the person who worked with him in prison did. But, Henry has stayed out of prison for some time and says he has maintained his sobriety. I would suggest that this outcome is the best you can get with ASPD addicts. In addition, it may not be the usual outcome that occurs. As was noted in the Preface, it was difficult to find ASPD case studies for people who weren't incarcerated. It was fortunate to get Rick's story before he re-offended.

The most important aspect of dealing with (the term "treatment" is probably not an accurate description of what is done with ASPD addicts) ASPD addicts is to provide certainty that the consequences of continuing their behavior will be much worse than the pleasure from continuing their behavior. ASPD addicts (at least some ASPD addicts) will modify their behavior if they know for certain that they will go back to prison if they have a dirty drug test or if they break the law. So, warnings, second chances, and threats that are not carried out are the absolute worst way to deal with an ASPD addict. Usually, the ASPD addict has to experience a rapid and severe consequence to get the message. Unfortunately, our criminal justice system is not organized this way. There can be long delays between actions and consequences and there is a tendency to try and keep people out of prison because of overcrowding and costs. As a result, ASPD addicts may believe (and be reinforced for this belief) that they can escape the consequences of their criminal activities and other inappropriate behavior.

When working with ASPD addicts, it is helpful to utilize a peer recovery support network of ex-offenders. These peers are harder to manipulate than professionals or recovering peers who are not ex-offenders. Ex-offender recovering peers who are not ASPD have had plenty of contact with ASPD addicts while in jail or prison and therefore, are knowledgeable in regard to the manipulative strategies and techniques they use. If a recovering peer is ASPD, there certainly is a danger that the individuals will collude and manipulate everyone. On the other hand, the ASPD recovering ex-offender is probably in the best position to clearly explain to the ASPD addict why it is in his best interest to stay out of trouble.

In terms of "counseling" strategies, there simply is no evidence that any of the known approaches are effective with this population. Delving into traumatic childhood histories, demonstrating unconditional positive regard, reframing cognitions, reinforcing positive behavior, and improving communication skills are all worthless. The message has to be pretty straightforward: "If you do this anymore, you will get locked up. The only way you can get your needs met is to stop (drinking, drugging, stealing, cheating, lying, or whatever). So, make a choice. Do you want to have fun for a limited amount of time and spend the rest of your time in prison or do you want to stay free but not be able to do everything you want to do?" But, if the first part of this dichotomy does not occur as threatened (i.e., getting locked up), this strategy won't work.

Regardless of how consistent the message is and in spite of follow-through on consequences, a whole lot of ASPD addicts will not change their behavior and incarceration is the only solution. In some cases, this is really clear from the start. I have conducted evaluations on some ASPD addicts who were really scary and I had no hope that they would change their behavior. But, the field of human behavior is not an exact science and we live in a society in which the suspicion of what you might do in the future is not a sufficient reason to keep you incarcerated (except for sexual offenders and suspected terrorists). So, everyone, even ASPD addicts, deserves at least one chance to change. Those who are not violent offenders may receive multiple chances. But, at some point, it is a waste of time and resources to continue to try and "treat" this population. If ASPD addicts keep breaking the law, we have a way to deal with them through the prison system. If we don't want to have the expense of incarceration in prison, I believe we should have residential drug-consumption facilities where these chronic ASPD addicts can use alcohol and other drugs (supplied by the facility) as long as all the drinking and drugging occurs at the facility and there is no violence. Any violation would result in prison. The risk of overdose could be managed by the distribution system. The residents would have to agree to a certain minimum length of stay and would only be released after a period of detoxification and abstinence.

I realize that the concept of residential drug-consumption facilities is too radical to be implemented in this country at this time. However, I do wish that policy makers, law enforcement and correction professionals, researchers, and treatment providers could engage in a frank discussion about ASPD addicts. Simply continuing with the current system of cycling these individuals through the criminal justice and treatment systems repeatedly is not working.

INTERVENTIONS FOR FUNCTIONAL ADDICTS

Considering the description and case studies of functional addicts, it would be reasonable to question the need for interventions with this group. After all, the individuals in this group are, by definition, functional. However, functional does not mean free of problems and, as illustrated in the case examples, these functional addicts have had difficulties in the past related to their alcohol and other drug use and may have problems in the future.

The major focus of interventions with functional addicts involves strategies designed to moderate alcohol and other drug use early in the process. When the different subtypes of addicts were discussed in Chapter 1, it was noted that the functional subtype had the highest average age (41) of any of the groups. Therefore, it is logical to assume that there are opportunities for professionals to intervene with people who are likely to become functional addicts before their alcohol and other drug use escalates. The interventions that would be applicable are called "screening, brief intervention and referral to treatment (SBIRT)" in the alcohol and other drug field.[5]

The rationale for SBIRT is that individuals who are heavy drinkers and frequent illicit drug users are the cause of significant problems (e.g., traffic accidents, work-place accidents) but may not have a substance use disorder. If these people can be convinced to moderate or stop their use of alcohol and other drugs, this will reduce the probability they will progress to a substance use disorder and the associated problems with these disorders (SBIRT is also used to identify people who may have a substance use disorder and refer them for assessment and treatment). SBIRT has primarily been implemented in health care settings (i.e., primary care offices, emergency rooms, community-based clinics) and normally involves a focus on alcohol use. However, the procedures can be easily adapted to include illicit drug use.

Since most people are used to completing forms about their health when they visit any type of health care setting, it is not difficult to include questions about substance use when a patient comes in to a primary care office, emergency room, or community clinic. The screening for alcohol problems can involve a couple of questions such as "How many days a week do you drink (on average)?"; "When you do drink, how many drinks do you usually have?"; and "What is the highest number of drinks you have had on any one day in the last month?" It can also include a short screening instrument. The most common questionnaire is called the Alcohol Use Disorders Identification Test (AUDIT), which is composed of 10 questions about alcohol use and the consequences of alcohol use. The patient responds to the frequency of each question on a five-point scale, with 0 being never and 5 being daily or very frequently. The cutoff scores for a problem with alcohol differ according to gender and age.

The National Institute on Alcohol Abuse and Alcoholism has published a guide for clinicians regarding suggested parameters for determining what constitutes problem drinking and recommendations for intervening with patients who drink too much.[6] For healthy men up to age 65, heavy drinking is defined as more than four drinks in a day and more than 14 drinks in a week. For healthy women and men over 65, it is more than three drinks in a day and more than 7 drinks in a week. If a patient can be classified as a heavy drinker based on these guidelines and/or a positive screening, the clinician is advised to do some additional assessment to determine if there is a likelihood of a substance use disorder, in which case the patient would be referred for a thorough assessment and possible treatment. If the patient is resistant to further screening or if the patient does not appear to have a substance use disorder, the clinician should provide the patient with information about his drinking level compared to the guidelines and possible consequences of continuing to drink at this level. The clinician should work with the patient on modifying his drinking and schedule follow up visits to monitor the patient's drinking.

Some of the specific interventions are dependent on the patient's readiness to change behavior. If a patient is totally resistant, it doesn't make much sense to try to develop a program to modify drinking. The best the clinician can do is to provide information and follow up the next time the patient is seen (if that is possible). A patient may be ambivalent about her drinking and open to considering what the clinician is saying. With this kind of patient, the clinician can offer some suggestions, express a willingness to discuss the patient's drinking at any time, and schedule a follow-up visit in the near future. Obviously, a patient who has considered the possibility that a drinking problem exists will be willing to work with the clinician on a plan of action.

SBIRT would be an effective intervention with those individuals who would probably become functional addicts if their alcohol and other drug use continued to progress. In a long-term study of problem drinkers, researchers found that two brief physician visits and two nurse follow-up phone calls resulted in reductions in number of drinks per week, binge drinking episodes, and frequency of excessive drinking compared to a control group. The results persisted over a 48-month period. The intervention group also had fewer days of hospitalization and emergency room visits.[7]

Another set of interventions for functional addicts that is related to SBIRT strategies is labeled "moderation management." These interventions involve cognitive and behavioral techniques of controlling alcohol and other drug use and include cognitive restructuring (i.e., changing thinking), behavioral contracts, contingency management (i.e., rewards and punishment for behavior), and drinking diaries. There is also a support group called "Moderation Management" to bring together individuals who prefer to continue to drink at some level as opposed to an abstinence-based program. Similar to Alcoholics Anonymous, Moderation Management Groups are free and run by nonprofessionals.

Moderation management is controversial in the substance abuse field. For those who subscribe to the disease model of addiction, moderation is not possible. From this perspective, if a person has the disease of addiction, the only way to manage the condition is to abstain from alcohol and other drugs. Most treatment providers do not believe that moderation management is possible. Because treatment providers only see those individuals with serious alcohol and other drug problems, their perspective is understandable. In addition, nearly every addict, regardless of the type, would like to continue to use alcohol and other drugs moderately. If an alternative to abstinence is presented to an addict, it will be almost always be preferred to abstinence. However, moderation management may be possible with functional addicts, especially if the interventions occur early in their alcohol and other drug history. Based on my own clinical experiences, it is very difficult for an individual with a long history of heavy alcohol and other drug use to successfully moderate their use over an extended period of time. It is much easier to have successful outcomes with relatively young (30- to 40-year-old) clients who have had few problems related to their alcohol and other drug use but who have become concerned about their level of drinking and/or drug use. In these cases, individuals may moderate their use of alcohol and other drugs and would never be classified as an addict.

CONCLUSION

This book is an effort to make the case for the existence of subtypes of addicts and for differentiating interventions and treatment based on subtypes. While I hope the argument is compelling, there is an issue that requires further exploration before I can expect the argument to be seriously considered.

In the case examples that have been presented, there were two disease model addicts who were alcoholics and did not discuss problems with other drugs. Clearly, these two individuals had extremely serious problems with alcohol. The two case examples of APSD addicts also had obvious problems, both with substances and with the law. Henry was addicted to methamphetamine and Rick primarily used alcohol and marijuana. In comparison, the functional addicts seem to be lightweights. George's substance use is limited to marijuana and occasional drinking. Mark does a variety of substances but seems to have the most problems with prescription pain pills. Amy is similar to Mark, although she seems to limiting her drug use to pain pills. Perhaps the difference between these cases has less to do with subtypes and more to do with the drugs the individuals use and the amount they use.

Of course, the differences in the amount of alcohol and other drugs the people in the cases use is one of the points of distinction between functional addicts and the other subtypes. We have hypothesized that functional addicts have a greater ability to control their alcohol and other drug use than do other addicts.

With regard to the types of drugs the individuals use, this is partially a function of the type of functional addict individuals who were willing to participate. For example, I tried to get an interview with a functional addict whose drug of choice is cocaine but the person was unwilling to participate. I could not successfully recruit a functional alcoholic to participate.

However, since alcohol is such a prominent substance in the stories of the two disease model addicts, I want to briefly describe my father, a classic functional addict. He has been dead for over 10 years now so I don't think any harm can come from talking about him. My father was a moderately successful small business owner who I remember as always going to work and being extremely reliable. He provided a comfortable living for our family. My parents were married for 52 years before he died. Although they had a tumultuous relationship, it did endure. My father was an uneducated man with good intelligence. He was gruff and obstinate but loving and affectionate with us. He always drank, every day. I never remember seeing him obviously drunk but he and my mother did fight about this drinking. He would go through a bottle of Seagram's VO whisky in about two days. I remember him being moody and irritable but never associated it with drinking. I wasn't ashamed to bring friends to the house and most of my friends found him amusing. At some point in early adulthood, I recognized that my father was an alcoholic and remember having discussions with my mother about it.

When Dad was about 65, he developed a respiratory illness and was hospitalized. The doctors diagnosed him with an ailment that required he be on a medication for one year that adversely impacted the liver. He was told that he could not drink any alcohol while on this medication. I told my mother to let the doctors know that dad was alcoholic because I was worried he would have a serious withdrawal syndrome from abruptly discontinuing his alcohol use. Of course, she didn't say anything. He stopped drinking that day and never drank again until he died, nearly 15 years later. He did not have any withdrawal. He didn't go to treatment or AA or anything else. I asked him later about why he decided not to drink anymore and he just said he didn't feel like it. He readily acknowledged his alcoholism.

As I have said on several occasions, one case doesn't prove a point. However, if you think that a person who only drinks alcohol cannot be a functional addict, you never met my father. He had a very high tolerance, never had significant behavior changes while intoxicated, managed his responsibilities during his drinking years, and was apparently able to control his alcohol use in situations where excessive drinking would be inappropriate. He was the definition of a functional addict.

The point is that the subtypes are real and that, as has been discussed, interventions and treatment have to account for these subtypes. Future research may identify other subtypes or discover differences between subtypes of alcoholics and subtypes of other addicts, although I have doubts about this. We clearly need to investigate why functional addicts are able to manage their alcohol and other drug use so differently than disease model addicts. The substance abuse field has evolved sufficiently to address these issues and the need for more effective interventions and treatment is a compelling reason to purse this type of investigation.

APPENDIX 1

Classification of Drugs[*]

Although there are different methods that are used to classify drugs, the most common scheme groups drugs by their pharmacological similarity. However, this scheme does not work well for "club drugs," which will be discussed as a separate classification. For each drug classification, there will be a description of the common drugs contained in the classification and some common street names, major effects, signs of intoxication, signs of overdose, tolerance, withdrawal, and acute and chronic effects. It should be noted that the term "drugs" includes both legal and illegal mood-altering substances.

CENTRAL NERVOUS SYSTEM DEPRESSANTS

Central nervous system (CNS) depressants (also referred to as sedative-hypnotics) depress the overall functioning of the central nervous system to induce sedation, drowsiness, and coma. The drugs in this classification include the most commonly used and abused psychoactive drug, alcohol; prescription drugs used for anxiety, sleep disturbance, and seizure control; and over-the-counter medications for sleep disturbance, colds and allergies, and coughs. In general, CNS depressants are extremely dangerous. There are approximately 79,000 deaths annually caused by excessive

*This information was adapted, with permission from Sage Publications, from G. L. Fisher, 2009. Drugs, classification of. In G. L. Fisher & N. A. Roget (Eds.). *Encyclopedia of Substance Abuse Prevention, Treatment, and Recovery* (pp. 330–339). Thousand Oaks, CA: Sage.

alcohol use in the United States, the third leading lifestyle cause of death.[1] Alcohol in combination with other drugs accounted for over one-quarter of drug abuse-related emergency room episodes in 2007.[2]

Drugs in This Classification. Alcohol is the most well-known CNS depressant because of its widespread use and legality. The alcohol content of common beverages is beer, 3% to 6%; wine, 11% to 20%; liqueurs, 25% to 35%; and liquor (whiskey, gin, vodka, etc.) 40% to 50%. Barbiturates are prescription drugs used to aid sleep for insomniacs and for the control of seizures. These drugs include Seconal (reds, red devils), Nembutal (yellows, yellow jackets), Tuinal (rainbows), Amytal (blues, blue heaven), and Phenobarbital. There are also nonbarbiturate sedative-hypnotics with similar effects but with different pharmacological properties. These include Doriden (goofballs), Quaalude (ludes), Miltown, and Equinil. The development of benzodiazepines, minor tranquilizers, reduced the number of prescriptions for barbiturates written by physicians. These drugs were initially seen as safe and having little abuse potential. Although the minor tranquilizers cannot be easily used in suicide as can barbiturates, the potential for abuse is significant. The benzodiazepines are among the most widely prescribed drugs and include Valium, Librium, Dalmane, Halcion, Xanax, and Ativan.

Finally, certain over-the-counter medications contain depressant drugs. Sleep aids such as Nytol and Sominex, cold and allergy products, and cough medicines may contain scopolamine, antihistamines, or alcohol to produce the desired effects.

Major Effects. The effects of CNS depressants are related to the dose, method of administration, and tolerance of the individual, factors that should be kept in mind as the effects are discussed. At low doses, these drugs produce a feeling of relaxation and calmness. They induce muscle relaxation, disinhibition, and a reduction in anxiety. Judgment and motor coordination are impaired, and there is a decrease in reflexes, pulse rate, and blood pressure. At high doses, the person demonstrates slurred speech, staggering, and, eventually, sleep. Phenobarbital and Valium have anticonvulsant properties and are used to control seizures. The benzodiazepines are also used to clinically control the effects from alcohol withdrawal.

Overdose. Alcohol overdose is common. We refer to this syndrome as being "drunk." The symptoms include staggering, slurred speech, extreme disinhibition, and blackouts (an inability to recall events that occurred when the individual was intoxicated). Generally, the stomach goes into spasm and the person will vomit, helping to eliminate alcohol from the body. However, the rapid ingestion of alcohol, particularly in a nontolerant individual, may result in coma and death. This happens most frequently with young people who participate in drinking contests. Because these drugs depress the central nervous system, overdose is extremely dangerous and can be fatal. Since the fatal dosage is only 10 to 15 times the therapeutic dosage, barbiturates are often used in suicides, which is one reason they are not frequently prescribed. It is far more difficult to overdose on the minor tranquilizers. However, CNS depressants have a synergistic, or potentiation, effect, meaning that the effect of a drug is enhanced as a result of the presence of another drug. For example, if a person has been drinking and then takes a minor tranquilizer such as Xanax, the effect of the Xanax may be dramatically enhanced. This combination has been the cause of many accidental deaths and emergency room visits.

Tolerance. There is a rapid development of tolerance to all CNS depressant drugs. Cross-tolerance also develops. This is another cause of accidental overdose. The tolerance to CNS depressants that develops is also one reason that the use of the minor tranquilizers has become problematic. People are given prescriptions to alleviate symptoms such as anxiety and sleep disturbance that are the result of other problems, such as marital discord. The minor tranquilizers temporarily relieve the symptoms but the real problem is never addressed. The person continues to use the drug to alleviate the symptoms, but tolerance develops and increasing dosages must be used to achieve the desired effect. This is a classic paradigm for the development of addiction and/or overdose.

Withdrawal. The withdrawal syndrome from CNS depressants can be medically dangerous. The symptoms may include anxiety, irritability, loss of appetite, tremors, insomnia, and seizures. In the severe form of alcohol withdrawal called delirium tremens (DTs), additional symptoms are fever, rapid heartbeat, and hallucinations. People can and do die from the withdrawal from CNS depressants. Therefore, the detoxification process for these drugs should include close supervision and the availability of medical personnel. Chronic, high-dosage users of these drugs should be discouraged from detoxifying without support and supervision. For detoxification in a medical setting, minor tranquilizers can be used, in decreasing dosages, to reduce the severity of the withdrawal symptoms.

Acute and Chronic Effects. In terms of damage to the human body and to society, alcohol is the most dangerous psychoactive drug (tobacco causes far more health damage). Alcohol has a damaging effect on every organ system. Chronic effects include permanent loss of memory, gastritis, esophagitis, ulcers, pancreatitis, cirrhosis of the liver, high blood pressure, weakened heart muscles, and damage to a fetus, including fetal alcohol syndrome. Other chronic effects include family, social, occupational, and financial problems. Acutely, alcohol is the cause of many traffic and other accidents and is involved in many acts of violence and crime. The yearly monetary cost to the United States attributable to alcohol is estimated to be nearly $200 billion.[3] Certainly, the other CNS depressants can cause the same kinds of both acute and chronic problems that are caused by alcohol abuse.

CENTRAL NERVOUS SYSTEM STIMULANTS

CNS stimulants affect the body in the opposite manner to the CNS depressants. These drugs increase respiration, heart rate, motor activity, and alertness. This classification includes highly dangerous, illegal substances such as crack cocaine, medically useful stimulants such as Ritalin, drugs with relatively minor psychoactive effects such as caffeine, and the most deadly drug habitually used, nicotine. The drugs in this classification were mentioned in 34% of the drug abuse-related emergency room episodes in 2007.[4]

Drugs in This Classification. Cocaine (coke, blow, toot, snow) and the freebase or smokeable forms of cocaine (crack, rock, base) are the most infamous of the CNS stimulants. Cocaine is found in the coca leaves of the coca shrub, which grows in Central and South America. The leaves are processed and produce coca paste. The paste is, in turn, processed to form the white hydrochloride salt powder most people know as cocaine. Of course, before it is sold on the street, it is adulterated or "cut" with substances such as powdered sugar, talc, arsenic, lidocaine, strychnine, or methamphetamine. Crack is produced by mixing the cocaine powder with baking soda and water and heating the solution. The paste that forms is hardened and cut into hard pieces or rocks. The mixing and heating process removes most of the impurities from the cocaine. Therefore, crack is a more pure form of cocaine than is cocaine hydrochloride salt powder. The vaporization point is lowered so the cocaine can be smoked, reaching the brain in one heartbeat less than if it is injected.

Amphetamines are also CNS stimulants, and one form in particular, methamphetamine, is a major drug of addiction. The amphetamines include Benzedrine (crosstops, black beauties), Methedrine or methamphetamine (crank, meth, crystal), and Dexedrine (dexies). There are also nonamphetamine stimulants with similar properties such as Ritalin and Cylert (used in the treatment of attention deficit-hyperactivity disorder) and Preludin (used in the treatment of obesity). Drugs in this classification are synthetic (not naturally occurring), and the amphetamines were widely prescribed in the 1950s and 1960s for weight control. Some forms of CNS stimulants are available without a prescription and are contained in many substances we use on a regular basis. Caffeine is found in coffee, teas, colas, and chocolate as well as in some over-the-counter products designed to help people stay awake (e.g., NoDoz, Alert, Vivarin). Phenyl-propanolamine is a stimulant found in appetite-control products sold over-the-counter (e.g., Dexatrim). These products are abused by individuals who chronically diet (e.g., anorexics). Although it has only mild euphoric properties, nicotine is the highly addictive stimulant drug found in tobacco products. According to the Centers for Disease Control and Prevention, an estimated 440,000 Americans die each year from smoking-related illnesses.[5]

Major Effects. The uses of CNS stimulants have an interesting history. As many people know, Sigmund Freud wrote the paper "Über Coca (1884)," which described the use of cocaine to treat a number of medical problems. Originally, Coca-Cola contained cocaine. In the 1980s, cocaine was depicted in the popular press as a relatively harmless drug. Amphet-amines were used in World War II to combat fatigue and were issued by the U.S. armed forces during the Korean War. These drugs have a long history of use by long-distance truck drivers, students cramming for exams, and women trying to lose weight. As with most of the psychoac-tive drugs, some of the CNS stimulants (cocaine and amphetamines) have a recreational use. The purpose is to "get high," or to experience a sense of euphoria. Amphetamine and cocaine users report a feeling of self-confidence and self-assurance. There is a "rush" that is experienced, par-ticularly when cocaine is smoked and when cocaine and methampheta-mine are injected. The high from amphetamines is generally less intense but longer acting than cocaine. CNS stimulants result in psychomotor stimulation, alertness, and elevation of mood. There is an increase in heart rate and blood pressure. Performance may be enhanced with increased activity level, one reason why athletes use CNS stimulants. These drugs also suppress appetite and combat fatigue. That's why people who want to lose weight and people who want to stay awake for long periods of time (e.g., truck drivers) use amphetamines.

Overdose. CNS stimulants activate the reward center of the brain. The most powerful of these drugs result in the body's not experiencing hunger, thirst, or fatigue. There is no built-in satiation point, so humans can continue using cocaine and amphetamines until there are no more or they die. Therefore, the compulsion to use, the desire to maintain the high, and the unpleasantness of withdrawal make overdose fairly common. There may be tremors, sweating and flushing, rapid heartbeat (tachycardia), anxiety, insomnia, paranoia, convulsions, heart attack, or stroke. Death from overdose has been widely publicized because it has occurred with some famous movie stars and athletes. However, far more people experience chronic problems from CNS stimulant addictions than from overdose reactions.

Tolerance. There is a rapid tolerance to the pleasurable effects of cocaine and amphetamines and the stimulating effects of tobacco and caffeine. If you drink five or six cups a day of combinations of coffee, tea, and colas, you probably know this with regard to caffeine. You will find that if you stop using caffeine for a couple of weeks and then start again, the initial doses of caffeine produce a minor "buzz," alertness, and/or restlessness. The rapid tolerance to the euphoric effects of cocaine and amphetamines leads to major problems with these drugs. The pleasurable effects are so rewarding, particularly when the drugs are smoked or injected, that the user is prone to compulsively use in an effort to recapture the euphoric effects. When injected or smoked, the effects are enhanced but of relatively short duration. Continual use to achieve the high leads to rapid tolerance. The user is then unable to feel the pleasure but must continue to use the drug to reduce the pain of withdrawal. A sensitization or reverse tolerance can occur, particularly with cocaine. In this instance, a chronic user with a high tolerance has an adverse reaction (i.e., seizure) to a low dose.

Withdrawal. Unlike the withdrawal from CNS depressants, the withdrawal from these drugs is not medically dangerous. However, it is extremely unpleasant. The withdrawal from cocaine and amphetamines is called "crashing." The severe symptoms usually last two to three days and include intense drug craving, irritability, depression, anxiety, and lethargy. However, the depression, drug craving, and an inability to experience pleasure may last for several months as the body chemistry returns to normal. Suicidal ideation and attempts are frequent during this time, as are relapses. Recovering cocaine and amphetamine addicts can become very discouraged with the slow rate of the lifting of depression, and, therefore, support is very important during this time.

Acute and Chronic Effects. As previously stated, the acute effects of CNS stimulants can be dramatic and fatal. These include heart attacks, strokes, seizures, and respiratory depression. However, the results of chronic use cause the most problems. The addictive properties of these drugs are extremely high. Individuals with addictions to cocaine and amphetamines spend a tremendous amount of money to obtain drugs, and they encounter serious life problems related to their addiction. Also, there is an increased risk of strokes and cardiovascular problems, depression, and suicide in chronic users. Symptoms of paranoid schizophrenia can occur. If cocaine or amphetamines are snorted, perforation of the nasal septum can occur. Injection of CNS stimulants has the same risks as injecting other drugs (e.g., hepatitis, HIV). Since these drugs suppress appetite, chronic users are frequently malnourished.

OPIOIDS

The opioids are naturally occurring (opium poppy extracts) and synthetic drugs that are commonly used for their analgesic (pain relief) and cough-suppressing properties. Opium was used by early Egyptian, Greek, and Arabic cultures for the treatment of diarrhea, since there is a constipating effect to this drug. Greek and Roman writers such as Homer and Virgil wrote of the sleep-inducing properties of opium, and recreational use of the drug in these cultures did occur. Morphine was isolated from opium in the early 1800s and was widely available without prescription until the early 1900s, when the nonmedical use of opioids was banned. Heroin accounted for 10% of drug abuse-related emergency room episodes for illicit drugs in 2007, while other opioids were involved in nearly half of emergency room visits for nonmedical pharmaceuticals.[6]

Drugs in This Classification. The opioids include opium, codeine, morphine, heroin (smack, horse), and buprenorphine, as well as familiar brand names such as Dilaudid (hydromorphone), OxyContin and Percocet (oxycodone), Loratab and Vicodin (hydrocodone), Darvocet (propoxyphene), Dolophine (methadone), and Demerol (meperidine). The Federal Drug Administration issued a recall for Propoxyphene on November 19, 2010 due to adverse side effects and it no longer will be available.

Major Effects. Opioids have medically useful effects, including pain, cough, and diarrhea suppression. Obviously, there is also a euphoric effect that accounts for the recreational use of these drugs. They can also produce nausea and vomiting and itching. They have a sedating effect, and the pupils of the eyes become constricted. Methadone, or Dolophine, is a synthetic opioid that does not have the dramatic euphoric effects of heroin, has a longer duration of action (12 to 24 hours compared with 3 to 6 hours for heroin), and blocks the symptoms of withdrawal when heroin is discontinued. This is the reason for the use of methadone in the treatment of opioid addiction. In the last few years, methadone in pill form is being frequently prescribed for pain relief. Buprenorphine (usually sold under the brand name Suboxone) is now being prescribed in an office setting to treat opioid dependence.

Overdose. Death from overdose of injectable opioids (usually heroin) can occur from the direct action of the drug on the brain, resulting in respiratory depression. Death can also occur from an allergic reaction to the drug or to substances used to cut it, possibly resulting in cardiac arrest. Overdose of other drugs in this classification may include symptoms such as slow breathing rate, decreased blood pressure, pulse rate, temperature, and reflexes. The person may become extremely drowsy and lose consciousness. There may be flushing and itching skin, abdominal pain, and nausea and vomiting. There has been a recent rise in overdose deaths resulting from the pill form of methadone. Methadone dissipates in the body much more slowly than other opioids. Users who have developed some tolerance may take doses more frequently than recommended because they are not experiencing the effects of methadone. However, the drug is still active in the body and this may result in an overdose.

Tolerance. Frequency of administration and dosage of opioids is related to the development of tolerance. Tolerance develops rapidly when the drugs are repeatedly administered but does not develop when there are prolonged periods of abstinence. The tolerance that does develop is to the euphoric, sedative, analgesic, and respiratory effects of the drugs. This tolerance results in the individual's administration of doses that would kill a nontolerant person. The tolerant individual becomes accustomed to using high doses, which accounts for death due to overdose in longtime opioid users who have been detoxified and then go back to using. Cross-tolerance to natural and synthetic opioids does occur. However, there is no cross-tolerance to CNS depressants. This fact is important, because the combination of moderate to high doses of opioids and alcohol or other CNS depressants can (and often does) result in respiratory depression and death.

Withdrawal. When these drugs are used on a continuous basis, there is a rapid development of physical dependence. Withdrawal symptoms are unpleasant and uncomfortable but are rarely dangerous. The symptoms are analogous to a severe case of the flu, with running eyes and nose, restlessness, goose bumps, sweating, muscle cramps or aching, nausea, vomiting, and diarrhea. There is significant drug craving. These symptoms rapidly dissipate when opioids are taken, which accounts for relapse when a person abruptly quits on his or her own ("cold turkey"). When the drugs are not immediately available to the dependent individual, the unpleasant withdrawal symptoms can also result in participation in criminal activities in order to purchase the drugs.

Acute and Chronic Effects. As we have already stated, there is an acute danger of death from overdose from injecting opioids, particularly heroin, and from frequent and large ingestion of opioids in pill form. Also, the euphoric effects of opioids rapidly decrease as tolerance increases, and, as this tolerance occurs, the opioid use is primarily to ward off the withdrawal symptoms. Compared with the chronic use of CNS depressants, chronic use of the drugs themselves is less dangerous to the body. However, the route of administration and the lifestyle associated with chronic opioid use clearly has serious consequences. Obviously, there is the risk of communicable disease from the sharing of needles during intravenous use of opioids. The lifestyle of heroin addicts often includes criminal activity to secure enough money to purchase heroin. Women may participate in prostitution, which adds the associated risks of diseases and violence. Nutrition is frequently neglected. However, those individuals who have been involved in methadone maintenance programs for long periods of time do not experience negative health consequences from the use of methadone (which is taken orally).

HALLUCINOGENS

Many of the hallucinogens are naturally occurring and have been used for thousands of years. Some have been (and are currently) used as sacraments in religious rites and have been ascribed with mystical and magical properties. Today, many types of hallucinogens are synthetically produced in laboratories. Some of the hallucinogens became very popular in the 1960s and 1970s, with a drop in use in the 1980s. Although there was a resurgence of use from 1992 to 2001 among youth, recent surveys have shown the lowest use of hallucinogens since the surveys were started in 1975.

Drugs in This Classification. This classification comprises a group of heterogeneous compounds. Although there may be some commonality in terms of effect, the chemical structures are quite different. The hallucinogens include LSD (acid, fry), psilocybin (magic mushrooms, shrooms), morning glory seeds (heavenly blue), mescaline (mesc, big chief, peyote), STP (serenity, tranquility, peace), and PCP (angel dust, hog). PCP is used as a veterinary anesthetic, primarily for primates.

Major Effects. These drugs produce an altered state of consciousness, including altered perceptions of visual, auditory, olfactory, and/or tactile senses and an increased awareness of inner thoughts and impulses. Sensory experiences may cross into one another (e.g., hearing color). Common sights and sounds may be perceived as exceptionally intricate and astounding. In the case of PCP, there may be increased suggestibility, delusions, and depersonalization and dissociation. Physiologically, hallucinogens produce a rise in pulse rate and blood pressure.

Overdose. With the exception of PCP, the concept of "overdose" is not applicable to the hallucinogens. "Bad trips" or panic reactions do occur and may include paranoid ideation, depression, undesirable hallucinations, and/or confusion. These are usually managed by providing a calm and supportive environment. An overdose of PCP may result in acute intoxication, acute psychosis, or coma. In the acute intoxication or psychosis, the person may be agitated, confused, and excited, and may exhibit a blank stare and violent behavior. Analgesia (insensibility to pain) occurs that may result in self-inflicted injuries and injuries to others when attempts are made to restrain the individual.

Tolerance. Tolerance to the hallucinogenic properties of these drugs occurs, as well as cross-tolerance between LSD and other hallucinogens. No cross-tolerance to cannabis (marijuana) has been demonstrated. Tolerance to PCP has not been demonstrated in humans.

Withdrawal. There is no physical dependence that occurs from the use of hallucinogens, although psychological dependence, including drug craving, does occur.

Acute and Chronic Effects. A fairly common and well-publicized adverse effect of hallucinogens is the experience of flashbacks. Flashbacks are the recurrence of the effects of hallucinogens long after the drug has been taken. Reports of flashbacks more than five years after taking a hallucinogen have been reported, although abatement after several months is more common. With regard to LSD, there are acute physical effects, including a rise in heart rate and blood pressure, higher body temperature, dizziness, and dilated pupils. Mental effects include sensory distortions, dreaminess, depersonalization, altered mood, and impaired concentration. "Bad trips" involve acute anxiety, paranoia, fear of loss of control, and delusions. Individuals with preexisting mental disorders may experience more severe symptoms. With regard to chronic effects, the rare but frightening experience of flashbacks has already been mentioned. On the other hand, PCP does result in significant adverse effects. Chronic use may result in psychiatric problems including depression, anxiety, and paranoid psychosis. Accidents, injuries, and violence occur frequently.

CANNABINOLS

Marijuana is the most widely used illegal drug. Over 18% of adults in the 18- to 25-year-old range reported using marijuana in the previous month.[7] The earliest references to the drug date back to 2700 BC. In the 1700s, the hemp plant (*Cannabis sativa*) was grown in the colonies for its fiber, which was used in rope. Beginning in 1926, states began to outlaw the use of marijuana because it was claimed to cause criminal behavior and violence. Marijuana use became popular with mainstream young people in the 1960s. Some states have basically decriminalized possession of small amounts of marijuana, although, according to the federal government, it remains a drug that has no medical uses and is extremely dangerous. Emergency room episodes in which marijuana was mentioned made up 16% of the total drug abuse-related emergency room visits in 2007.[8]

Drugs in This Classification. The various cannabinols include marijuana (grass, pot, weed, joint, reefer, dube), hashish, charas, bhang, ganja, and sinsemilla. The active ingredient is delta-9-tetrahydrocannabinol (THC). Hashish and charas have a THC content of 7% to 14%; ganja and sinsemilla, 4% to 7%; and bhang and marijuana, 2% to 5%. However, recent improvements in growing processes have increased the THC content of marijuana sold on the street. For simplicity, the various forms of cannabinols will be referred to as "marijuana."

Major Effects. Marijuana users experience euphoria; enhancement of taste, touch, and smell; relaxation; increased appetite; altered time sense; and impaired immediate recall. An enhanced perception of the humor of situations or events may occur. The physiological effects of marijuana include increase in pulse rate and blood pressure, dilation of blood vessels in the cornea (which produces bloodshot eyes), and dry mouth. Motor skills and reaction time are slowed. Marijuana may be medically useful in reducing nausea and vomiting from chemotherapy, stimulating appetite in AIDS and other wasting-syndrome patients, treating spasticity and nocturnal spasms complicating multiple sclerosis and spinal cord injury, controlling seizures, and managing neuropathic pain. However, further clinical studies are necessary to reach conclusions on the value of marijuana in medical treatment.

Overdose. Overdose is unusual because the normal effects of marijuana are not enhanced by large doses. Intensification of emotional responses and mild hallucinations can occur, and the user may feel "out of control." As with hallucinogens, many reports of overdose are panic reactions to the normal effects of the drug. In individuals with preexisting mental disorders (e.g., schizophrenia), high doses of marijuana may exacerbate symptoms such as delusions, hallucinations, disorientation, and depersonalization.

Tolerance. Tolerance is a controversial area with regard to marijuana. The difference of opinion as to whether tolerance develops slowly or quickly may be due to type of subject studied and various definitions of "dosage." For example, tolerance rapidly occurs in animals but only with frequent use of high doses in humans. At the very least, chronic users probably become accustomed to the effects of the drug and are experienced in administering the proper dosage to produce the desired effects. Cross-tolerance to CNS depressants, including alcohol, has been demonstrated.

Withdrawal. A withdrawal syndrome can be observed in chronic, high-dosage users who abruptly discontinue their use. The symptoms include irritability, restlessness, decreased appetite, insomnia, tremor, chills, and increased body temperature. The symptoms usually last three to five days.

Acute and Chronic Effects. Marijuana has been and continues to be controversial. Ballot measures in several states have involved marijuana laws. This controversy is related to the facts and myths regarding marijuana's acute and chronic effects. The professional community has as many views of the "facts" regarding marijuana as does the general public. However, marijuana should clearly not be among the most dangerous drugs (such as heroin, cocaine, and methamphetamine) on federal government schedules, although no psychoactive drug is safe. Marijuana can and does result in significant life problems for many people. If death is the measure of dangerousness, marijuana is not acutely or chronically dangerous. However, the effect on motor skills and reaction time certainly impairs the user's ability to drive a car, boat, plane, or other vehicle, and marijuana use has also been detected in a significant number of victims of vehicle and nonvehicle accidents. Chronic use of marijuana does seem to have an adverse effect on lung function, although there is no direct evidence that it causes lung cancer. Although an increase in heart rate occurs, there does not seem to be an adverse effect on the heart. As is the case with CNS depressants, marijuana suppresses the immune system. Chronic marijuana use decreases the male hormone testosterone (as does alcohol) and adversely affects sperm formation. However, no effect on male fertility or sexual potency has been noted. Female hormones are also reduced, and impairment in ovulation has been reported.

INHALANTS AND VOLATILE HYDROCARBONS

Inhalants and volatile hydrocarbons consist largely of chemicals that can be legally purchased and that are normally used for nonrecreational purposes. In addition, this classification includes some drugs that are used legally for medical purposes. As psychoactive drugs, most of these substances are used mainly by young people, particularly in low socioeconomic areas. Since most of these chemicals are accessible in homes and are readily available for purchase, they are easily used as psychoactive drugs by young people who are beginning drug experimentation and by individuals who are unable to purchase other mind-altering substances due to finances or availability.

Drugs in This Classification. The industrial solvents and aerosol sprays that are used for psychoactive purposes include gasoline, kerosene, chloroform, airplane glue, lacquer thinner, acetone, nail polish remover, model cement, lighter fluid, carbon tetrachloride, fluoride-based sprays, and metallic paints. Volatile nitrites are amyl nitrite (poppers), butyl and isobutyl (locker room, rush, bolt, quick silver, zoom). Amyl nitrite has typically been used in the gay community. In addition, nitrous oxide (laughing gas), a substance used by dentists, is also included in this classification.

Major Effects. The solvents and sprays reduce inhibition and produce euphoria, dizziness, slurred speech, an unsteady gait, and drowsiness. Nystagmus (constant involuntary movements of the eyes) may be noted. The nitrites alter consciousness and enhance sexual pleasure. The user may experience giddiness, headaches, and dizziness. Nitrous oxide produces giddiness, a buzzing or ringing in the ears, and a sense that the user is about to pass out.

Overdose. Overdose of these substances may produce hallucinations, muscle spasms, headaches, dizziness, loss of balance, irregular heartbeat, and coma from lack of oxygen.

Tolerance. Tolerance does develop to nitrous oxide but does not seem to develop to the other inhalants.

Withdrawal. There does not appear to be a withdrawal syndrome associated with these substances.

Acute and Chronic Effects. The most critical acute effect of inhalants is a factor of the method of administration, which can result in loss of consciousness, coma, or death from lack of oxygen. Respiratory arrest, cardiac arrhythmia, or asphyxiation may occur. Many of these substances are highly toxic, and chronic use may cause damage to the liver, kidneys, brain, and lungs.

CLUB DRUGS

Rather than sharing pharmacological similarities, the drugs that will be discussed in this section are grouped together because of the environment in which they are commonly used. The use of these drugs is primarily by youth and young adults associated with dance clubs, bars, and all-night dance parties ("raves"). It would not make sense to discuss the common characteristics of overdose, tolerance, withdrawal, and acute and chronic effects since the drugs are not related pharmacologically. However, it is important to reference these drugs as a separate class because of the wide media coverage of club drugs. The most appropriate pharmacological classification for each drug will be referenced.

Rohypnol (roofies) is a benzodiazepine (CNS depressant) that is illegal in the United States, but widely prescribed in Europe as a sleeping pill. When used in combination with alcohol, Rohypnol produces disinhibition and amnesia. Rohypnol has become known as the "date rape" drug because of reported instances in which women have been unknowingly given the drug while drinking and then sexually assaulted, after which they cannot easily remember the events surrounding the incident. MDMA (ecstasy) has the properties of both the CNS stimulants and hallucinogens. It is taken in tablet form primarily, but can also be found in powder and liquid forms. It is relatively inexpensive and long lasting. The euphoric effects include rushes of exhilaration and the sensation of understanding and accepting others. Some people experience nausea, and depression may be experienced following use. Deaths have been reported from ecstasy use primarily as a result of severe dehydration from dancing for long periods of time without drinking water. Ecstasy can be used compulsively and become psychologically addictive. Ketamine (K or special K) is generally considered to be a hallucinogen. It is used as a veterinary anesthetic and is usually cooked into a white powder from its liquid form and snorted. The euphoric effect of ketamine involves dissociative anesthetics or separating perception from sensation. Users report feeling "floaty" or outside their body. Higher doses expand this experience. They may have some numbness in extremities. Ketamine is very dangerous in combination with depressants, since higher doses depress respiration and breathing. Frequent use may lead to mental disorders due to the hallucinogenic properties of the drug. Psychological dependence also occurs in frequent users. GHB (gamma hydroxybutyrate) is actually a synthetic steroid originally sold over the counter in health food stores as a body-building aid. GHB is usually sold as an odorless liquid that has a slight salty taste. The effects are similar to CNS depressants, with low doses resulting in euphoria, relaxation, and a feeling of happiness. However, higher doses can cause dizziness, drowsiness, vomiting, muscle spasms, and loss of consciousness. Overdoses can result in coma or death, as can mixing GHB with other CNS depressants such as alcohol. Physical dependence can occur. Other drugs, such as LSD, PCP, mescaline, and marijuana are sometimes classified as club drugs. However, since these drugs have a wider use, they have been discussed in other drug classifications.

APPENDIX 2

Treatment Approaches and Strategies[*]

INTRODUCTION

Alcohol and other drug treatment approaches and strategies are dependent upon the model of addiction adopted by the particular treatment program. However, there is a growing trend toward more eclectic approaches to treatment that combine aspects of different treatment models. While this is certainly good practice, it has also be driven by financial concerns, particularly in for-profit treatment programs. For example, some insurance companies pay for substance abuse treatment only if there is another mental disorder as well. This consideration has resulted in treatment programs developing "co-occurring disorders" programs and using components from a variety of treatment approaches.

Although it would be expected that all treatment programs utilize evidence-based practices (i.e., approaches and strategies validated by research), this is not always the case. Therefore, the treatment approaches and strategies described below are not necessarily "evidence-based" but are those most often used in both public sector and private substance abuse treatment programs.

---

*This information was adapted, with permission from Sage Publications, from G. L. Fisher, 2009. Treatment Approaches and Strategies. In G. L. Fisher & N. A. Roget (Eds.). *Encyclopedia of Substance Abuse Prevention, Treatment, and Recovery*. (pp. 936–941). Thousand Oaks, CA: Sage.

TREATMENT APPROACHES

Minnesota Model

Perhaps the most well-known and widely emulated approach to treatment is the Minnesota Model, developed by the Hazeldon Foundation in the 1940s and 1950s. The philosophy of the Minnesota Model can be described by four components. The first is the belief that patients can change attitudes, beliefs, and behaviors. Famous people who have completed the program, such as Betty Ford, Elizabeth Taylor, and Anthony Hopkins, are used as models to illustrate this belief. Second, the Minnesota Model adheres to the disease model of addiction. The term chemical dependency is preferred to addiction or alcoholism and is seen as a physical, psychological, social, and spiritual illness. The major characteristics of the disease model are taught. That is, chemical dependency is seen as a primary disease that is chronic, progressive, and potentially fatal. The focus of treatment is the disease and not secondary characteristics. The third philosophical component is illustrated by the long-term treatment goals of the Minnesota Model: abstinence from all mood-altering chemicals and improvement of lifestyle. Patients are not considered cured because the disease is believed to be incurable. However, through abstinence and personal growth, a chemically dependent individual can be in the process of recovery. Finally, the Minnesota Model uses the principles of Alcoholics Anonymous (AA) and Narcotics Anonymous (NA) in treatment, implying a heavy spiritual component to treatment.

The continuum of care includes assessment and diagnosis, detoxification, inpatient services, therapeutic communities, halfway houses, outpatient services, and aftercare. Group therapy is used and is concerned with present and future behavior as opposed to past causal factors. Groups are often confrontational. The family also receives therapy. Didactic experiences, including lectures and videotapes, are used to educate patients about the disease of chemical dependency and the consequences of the disease. Although the staff is composed of professionals from a number of disciplines (physicians, social workers, psychologists, nurses, and clergy), recovering addicts and alcoholics are also used as counselors. Patients have reading and writing assignments, such as reading the AA Twelve Steps and Twelve Traditions and writing their life histories. Attendance at AA/NA meetings is required, and patients are expected to work through the first three to five steps of AA while in treatment. There may also be work assignments and recreational activities, depending on the treatment setting. Aftercare includes attendance at AA or NA.

Behavioral Approaches

In contrast to the disease model of treatment exemplified by the Minnesota Model, behavioral models of treatment use techniques of classical and operant conditioning in the treatment of alcohol and other drug problems. Perhaps the best-known behavioral technique applied to alcohol problems is aversive conditioning, which is designed to reduce or eliminate the patient's desire for alcohol or drugs by pairing unpleasant stimuli or images with substances. The unpleasant stimuli most widely used are nausea, apnea (paralysis of breathing), electric shock, and various images. Nausea is the oldest and most commonly used of these stimuli, with fairly wide use in the former Soviet Union and in certain hospitals in the United States. The process is to give the patient a drug that, when combined with alcohol, produces severe nausea. In a supervised setting, the patient is then allowed to drink. In the classical conditioning paradigm, the feeling of severe nausea should quickly become associated with drinking alcohol. Electric shock can also be administered when the patient drinks, or a drug can be administered that produces apnea when alcohol is consumed. Since these procedures are painful, stressful, and potentially dangerous, careful screening of patients and medical supervision is necessary. Although electric shock can be used in the treatment of addiction to drugs other than alcohol, most references to aversive conditioning are related to the treatment of alcoholism.

Covert sensitization has major advantages over other forms of aversive conditioning techniques. This process involves pairing the consumption of the drug of choice with aversive images, such as nausea or negative consequences of alcohol or other drug use. The advantages are quite obvious. Since the patient does not actually experience nausea, electric shock, or apnea, there are no medical dangers. Therefore, patients would also be less likely to discontinue treatment.

Additional behavioral techniques have been used in treatment. Contingency contracting has been used where patients make monetary deposits that are forfeited if the patient does not complete the treatment program. Behavioral self-control training involves goal setting, self-monitoring, managing consumption, rewarding goal attainment, analyzing drinking situations, and learning coping skills. These techniques have been used to achieve abstinence or controlled use.

Another form of a behavioral approach to treatment is the community reinforcement approach (CRA). Although there are a variety of "twists" to this approach, the basic idea is to provide tangible rewards for achieving successful treatment goals. For example, CRA was applied in a 24-week outpatient program for cocaine addicts. For each "clean" urine sample, patients were given vouchers for retail goods that increased in value with consecutive cocaine-free samples.[1]

Pharmacological Approaches

Pharmacological procedures are also used in treatment. However, it is rare to find these procedures as the only intervention. Rather, they are usually used in conjunction with other treatment methods. The philosophy of treatment and the treatment setting may also determine whether drugs are used to treat alcohol and other drug problems. Treatment programs in nonhospital settings without medical staff obviously should not use drugs in treatment.

Detoxification, the period of time in which a patient is withdrawing from alcohol or other drugs, is frequently a time when medication is used. In the past, this process occurred in an inpatient, hospital setting. However, outpatient detoxification is now a common practice due to the high costs of hospitalization. In the detoxification process for alcohol and other central nervous system depressants, minor tranquilizers such as Valium or Xanax are often used to reduce the danger of seizures and the other uncomfortable and dangerous withdrawal symptoms. Careful medical supervision with a gradually decreasing dosage is necessary, since these minor tranquilizers are in the same drug classification as alcohol. Methadone is widely known for its use in treating opioid addiction. Methadone is a synthetic narcotic with a longer duration of effect than heroin, and ingestion blocks the euphoric effects of opioids. Once a patient is stabilized on a particular dose, he or she takes it to reduce or eliminate any withdrawal symptoms from heroin abstinence. The patient usually must visit a methadone clinic to receive the dose. Once a patient is stabilized on methadone, he or she can function normally. A new medication has been approved for use in treating opioid addiction, buprenorphine, an opioid that has proved to be as effective as methadone. The advantages of buprenorphine are that it is taken in tablet form, daily doses do not appear to be necessary, and it has relatively mild withdrawal symptoms. In the pill form administered to opioid addicts, naloxone is added to buprenorphine. The naloxone decreases the likelihood of abuse, because it blocks the "high" that could be achieved by injecting opioids. In addition, buprenorphine can be administered by general physicians in outpatient clinics, rather than in specialty clinics, as is the case with methadone. The approval of buprenorphine by the Federal Drug Administration has greatly increased the access to opioid-agonist treatment (i.e., using other opioid drugs) for heroin addicts. Antabuse (disulfiram) has been used in conjunction with other forms of alcohol treatment. When Antabuse is taken and alcohol is ingested during the following 24- to 48-hour period, the patient experiences facial flushing, heart palpitations and rapid heart rate, difficulty in breathing, nausea, and vomiting. Since Antabuse takes 30 minutes to work after ingestion, it has been of limited value in aversive conditioning. The patient must take Antabuse on a daily basis, and this raises an issue of the need for such medication. If an individual were motivated to take Antabuse daily, it would seem that he or she would probably be motivated to remain abstinent without Antabuse. However, some alcoholics, when tempted to use alcohol, are comforted by the fact that Antabuse will result in an unpleasant reaction if they drink. This awareness often reduces or eliminates the urge to use. Patients who use Antabuse must be warned against using over-the-counter products that contain alcohol, since the Antabuse will cause a reaction from the use of these products. There has been considerable publicity on the use of naltrexone in alcoholism treatment. Naltrexone is an opioid antagonist (i.e., a drug that blocks the effects of other opioids). However, it has also been found to reduce the craving for alcohol. Therefore, it is recommended as one strategy in a comprehensive treatment program, but not as the only strategy.

Other Approaches

The National Institute on Alcohol Abuse and Alcoholism (NIAAA) has developed treatment manuals for three very different approaches to alcohol treatment. The manuals were used in a large-scale study to investigate the effects of matching patients to treatment approaches. The first approach is called Twelve-Step Facilitation Therapy and is based on the principles of Alcoholics Anonymous. The treatment protocol familiarizes patients with the AA philosophy and encourages participation in AA. This approach is similar to the Minnesota Model. The second manual is called *Cognitive-Behavioral Therapy* and is based on a social-learning theory model. Skills to avoid relapse are taught. The third approach is called Motivational Enhancement Therapy and is designed to help patients identify and utilize personal resources to effect change. This approach is based on motivational psychology and is related to Motivational Interviewing.

TREATMENT STRATEGIES

The strategies that are used in treatment vary depending upon the approach of the treatment program and the treatment setting (e.g., outpatient or residential). Not all of these strategies are (or should be) applied to every patient. A treatment plan must be developed that is individualized according to the needs of the patient. The following are the most widely used strategies.

Individual, Group, and Family Counseling. The frequency, intensity, and approach to individual counseling varies widely between treatment programs. This is dependent on the staffing model of the treatment program and the credentials of the professional staff. Thus, a treatment program that employs mainly addiction counselors who are not trained at the master's level limits the types of issues that can be addressed in individual counseling and the philosophical orientations that are used. Obviously, programs employing master's and doctoral level addiction counselors and other mental health professionals can offer more extensive individual counseling services.

Traditionally, group counseling is often the primary approach of both residential and outpatient treatment programs. However, in many treatment programs, group counseling may actually be a confrontation of individuals in the group who are not "working the program," or it may simply be dissemination of educational information. It would be more useful for group work to help to develop concrete usable skills and to rehearse these behaviors in the group. In addition, such group counseling can be used to analyze drinking and drug-taking behaviors and to develop methods of coping, problem solving, and assertiveness, rather than being focused on gaining patient compliance to admit to having a disease. There has been an increasing use of family counseling in treatment programs. As with group counseling, what is sometimes called family counseling is actually education about the disease model and the family's role in the disease process. However, family counseling is an essential component of treatment. Clearly, the family system can serve to support or sabotage recovery, and addiction almost always creates significant problems within families. However, it is essential that family counseling be conducted by qualified mental health professionals.

Support Groups. While support groups should not be considered a treatment "strategy," they are so frequently a part of traditional treatment programs that they must be mentioned. The use of Twelve Step meetings as a treatment strategy and the utilization of the Twelve Step philosophy in treatment programs are consistent with the disease model of addiction and thus, are a central component of treatment programs utilizing the Minnesota Model.

While AA and NA are usually recommended for the alcoholic/addict, family members are encouraged to attend either Al-Anon (for intimate partners or relatives of addicts) or Alateen (for adolescent children of addicts) meetings. This is to introduce family members to the potential support available through Al-Anon or Alateen while the patient is still in treatment. Patients and family members may also be referred to ACOA (Twelve Step support for adult children of alcoholics) or CODA (Twelve Step support for codependent). There are alternative support groups to those that use the Twelve Step model. However, the acceptance of these alternatives in disease model treatment programs may be resisted.

Lifestyle Changes. Irrespective of the orientation of the treatment program, treatment strategies designed to bring about changes in the lifestyle of the patient are essential. For example, if patients return to the same friends and activities that were a part of their lives prior to treatment, relapse is highly probable. The range of lifestyle changes that must be addressed illustrates the complexity of comprehensive treatment and the need for long-term interventions for addicted individuals. The lifestyle areas that need to receive attention for a particular patient should be determined during assessment and should then be included in the treatment plan. The issue of friends, lovers, family members, and acquaintances is a focus of treatment. If a patient has close associations with individuals who use alcohol or other drugs, some difficult and painful decisions must be made. These topics may be discussed in individual, group, and family counseling. In addition, patients may need assistance with social skills in order to enhance their ability to make new friends. Many addicted individuals have relied on the use of alcohol and other drugs to feel comfortable in social situations and/or as a common bond to those with whom they spend time. The difficulty of this particular area can often be clearly illustrated with an adolescent who is told during treatment to avoid contact with friends who use. The adolescent returns to school after treatment and perceives his options as returning to a previous social group or having no friends at all. If relapse is to be avoided, the adolescent who is treated for an alcohol or other drug problem clearly needs continued support and assistance to help develop a new social group.

Since many individuals with substance abuse problems have used these substances to avoid negative emotions or to manage stress and pain, alternative methods of dealing with common life problems must also be taught in treatment. Strategies may involve stress-management techniques, relaxation procedures, and assertiveness training. The intent of such training is to provide the patient with skills to use in situations or in response to situations in which alcohol or other drug use was previously the only perceived option available. If the patient is not taught alternative methods for managing stress and tension, along with techniques to relax that do not involve drugs, relapse is a predictable response. Other lifestyle areas that may be a focus of intervention include vocational and educational planning, financial planning, living environment, and nutrition

Education. Many treatment programs, particularly those using a disease model, use lectures and films to provide patients with information on the disease model, on family issues, and on the social, medical, and psychological consequences of alcohol and other drug use. Although the teaching of educational information is a commonly used strategy in treatment, there is no evidence that providing information to addicts changes their behavior. However, as part of a comprehensive treatment program, it certainly makes sense to provide information to patients and family members. But education and information dissemination should not be expected to produce miraculous changes and, therefore, these activities should not be conducted at the expense of more useful treatment strategies.

Aftercare. For those individuals who enter treatment, recovery can be conceptualized as a three-stage process. The first stage is formal treatment, the second stage is aftercare, and the third stage is ongoing recovery. Aftercare refers to the interventions and strategies that will be implemented after formal treatment is completed. However, it more accurately should be called "continuing care," since aftercare programs are usually continuations of many of the strategies from formal treatment. The focus should be on the issues that require attention following discharge from formal treatment.

APPENDIX 3

Resources

I. Federal Agencies Related to Addiction Research and Treatment
  A. National Institute on Alcohol Abuse and Alcoholism: http://www.niaaa.nih.gov/AboutNIAAA/Pages/default.aspx
  B. National Institute on Drug Abuse: http://drugabuse.gov/nidahome.html
  C. Substance Abuse and Mental Health Services Administration, Center for Substance Abuse Treatment: http://csat.samhsa.gov/
II. Selected University Centers Related to Addiction Research, Policy, and Treatment
  A. The National Center on Addiction and Substance Abuse at Columbia University: http://www.casacolumbia.org/templates/Home.aspx?articleid=287&zoneid=32
  B. Center for the Application of Substance Abuse Technologies at the University of Nevada, Reno: http://casat.unr.edu/
  C. Center for Alcohol and Addiction Studies at Brown University: http://www.caas.brown.edu/
  D. UCLA Integrated Substance Abuse Programs: http://www.uclaisap.org/
III. Selected Reading
  A. W. White, 1998. *Slaying the dragon: The history of addiction treatment and recovery in America*. Bloomington, IL: Chestnut Health Systems/Lighthouse Institute. Comprehensive historical review of treatment written by a leading recovery advocate.

B. E. M. Jellinek, 1960. *The disease concept of alcoholism.* New Haven, CT: Hillhouse Press. The original book by the individual credited with developing the disease model of addiction.

C. National Institute on Drug Abuse, 2010. Drugs, Brains, and Behavior: The Science of Addiction. http://www.drugabuse.gov/scienceofaddiction/. This site, sponsored by the federal agency responsible for research on illicit drugs, uses understandable language and visual aids to explain the neurobiology of addiction.

D. A. T. McLellan, D. C. Lewis, C. P. O'Brien, & H. D. Kleber, 2000. Drug dependence: a chronic, medical illness: Implications for treatment, insurance, and outcome evaluation. *Journal of the American Medical Association* 284: 1689–1695. The journal article that made the case that addiction is a chronic medical condition by comparing addiction to other chronic conditions such as diabetes and hypertension.

E. H. B. Moss, C. M. Chen, & H. Yi, 2007. Subtypes of alcohol dependence in a nationally representative sample. *Drug and Alcohol Dependence* 91: 149–158. The report of the research conducted by the National Institute on Alcohol Abuse and Alcoholism scholars that identified the subtypes of alcoholics.

F. Center for Substance Abuse Treatment, 2005. *Substance abuse treatment for persons with co-occurring disorders.* Treatment Improvement Protocol (TIP) Series 42. DHHS Publication No. (SMA) 05-3992. Rockville, MD: Substance Abuse and Mental Health Services Administration. http://store.samhsa.gov/product/SMA08-3992. A free federal publication on the prevalence of various mental disorders that occur in patients with substance use disorders and the treatment implications of working with these patients.

G. G. L. Fisher, 2006. *Rethinking our war on drugs: Candid talk about controversial issues*, Chapter Seven, Controversial Issues in Treatment (pp. 125–145). Westport, CT: Praeger. In a book critiquing the "War on Drugs," this chapter focuses on the problems in the treatment system.

H. National Institute on Alcohol Abuse and Alcoholism, 2005. *Helping patients who drink too much: A clinician's guide.* NIH Publication No. 07-3769. http://pubs.niaaa.nih.gov/publications/practitioner/cliniciansguide2005/clinicians_guide.htm. A free publication designed for healthcare providers that provides simple-to-follow guidelines for identifying heavy drinkers and intervening with them.

I. Mid-Atlantic Addiction Technology Transfer Center, 2010. Motivational Interviewing: Resources for Clinicians, Researchers, and Trainers. http://www.motivationalinterview.org/. A federally sponsored site for clinicians interested in using motivational interviewing.

Notes

CHAPTER 1

1. Office of Applied Studies, Substance Abuse and Mental Health Services Administration, 2010. National Survey on Drug Use & Health. http://oas.samhsa.gov/NSDUH/2k9NSDUH/2k9ResultsP.pdf (accessed December 10, 2010).

2. *Ibid.*

3. American Psychiatric Association, 2000. *Diagnostic and statistical manual of mental disorders* (Fourth Edition, Text Revision). Washington, DC: American Psychiatric Association, p. 199.

4. *Ibid.*, p. 197.

5. G. L. Fisher, 2006. *Rethinking our war on drugs: Candid talk about controversial issues.* Westport, CT: Praeger, p. 10.

6. Center on Substance Abuse and Addiction, 2009. New CASA Report Finds Federal, State and Local Governments Spend Almost Half a Trillion Dollars a Year on Substance Abuse and Addiction. Press Release. http://www.casacolumbia.org/absolutenm/templates/PressReleases.aspx?articleid=556&zoneid=66 (accessed November 18, 2009).

7. S. Belenko, N. Patapis, & M. T. French, 2005. *Economic benefits of drug treatment: A critical review of the evidence for policy makers.* University of Pennsylvania: Treatment Research Institute.

8. Office of Applied Studies, Substance Abuse and Mental Health Services Administration, 2009. Treatment Episode Data Set (TEDS) 2006: Discharges from Substance Abuse Treatment Services. Table 2.3b: Discharges in 2006 by State and reason for discharge: TEDS 2006 percent

distribution. http://wwwdasis.samhsa.gov/teds06/tedsd2k6_508.pdf (accessed November 17, 2009).

9. Office of Applied Studies, Substance Abuse and Mental Health Services Administration, 2009. Treatment Episode Data Set (TEDS) 2006: Discharges from Substance Abuse Treatment Services. Table 2.6: Discharges in 2006 by characteristics at admissions and type of service: TEDS 2006 percent distribution of characteristics of admission. http://wwwdasis.samhsa.gov/teds06/tedsd2k6_508.pdf (accessed November 17, 2009).

10. Office of Applied Studies, Substance Abuse and Mental Health Services Administration, 2010. National Survey on Drug Use & Health. http://oas.samhsa.gov/NSDUH/2k9NSDUH/2k9ResultsP.pdf (accessed December 10, 2010).

11. *Ibid.*

12. E. M. Jellinek, 1960. *The disease model of addiction.* New Haven, CT: Hillhouse Press.

13. L. Leggio, G. A. Kenna, M. Fenton, E. Bonenfant, & R. M. Swift, 2009. Typologies of alcohol dependence. From Jellinek to genetics and beyond. *Neuropsychology Review* 19: 115–129.

14. H. B. Moss, C. M. Chen, & H. Yi, 2007. Subtypes of alcohol dependence in a nationally representative sample. *Drug and Alcohol Dependence* 91: 149–158.

15. *Ibid.*, p. 150.

CHAPTER 2

1. J. Frey, 2003. *A million little pieces.* New York: Anchor Books.

2. E .M. Jellinek, 1960. *The disease model of addiction.* New Haven, CT: Hillhouse Press.

3. E. Kurtz, 1990. *Not-God: A history of alcoholics anonymous.* Center City, MN: Hazelton.

4. J. E. Royce, 1989. *Alcohol problems and alcoholism: A comprehensive survey* (Rev. ed.). New York: The Free Press.

5. E. M. Jellinek, 1952. Phases of alcohol addiction. *Quarterly Journal of Studies on Alcohol* 13: 673–684, 682.

6. *Ibid.*

7. J. E. Royce, 1989. *Alcohol problems and alcoholism: A comprehensive survey* (Rev. ed.). New York: The Free Press.

8. *Ibid.*

9. D. L. Ohlms, 1983. *The disease concept of alcoholism.* Belleville, IL: Gary Whiteaker Corporation, p. 5.

10. T. E. Bratter, 1985. Special clinical psychotherapeutic concerns for alcoholic and drug addicted individuals. In T. E. Bratter &

G. G. Forrest (Eds.). *Alcoholism and substance abuse: Strategies for clinical intervention* (pp. 523–574). New York: The Free Press.

11. D. A. Ward, 1990. Conceptions of the nature and treatment of alcoholism. In D.A. Ward (Ed.). *Alcoholism: Introduction to theory and treatment* (pp. 4–16). Dubuque, IA: Kendall/Hunt Publishing.

12. J. E. Royce, 1989. *Alcohol problems and alcoholism A comprehensive survey* (Rev. ed.). New York: The Free Press.

13. *Ibid.*, p. 132.

14. J. C. McCarthy, 1988. The concept of addictive disease. In D. E. Smith & D. R. Wesson (Eds.). *Treating cocaine dependency* (pp. 21–30). Minneapolis, MN: Hazeldon.

15. A. T. McLellan, D. C. Lewis, C. P. O'Brien, & H. D. Kleber, 2000. Drug dependence: a chronic, medical illness: Implications for treatment, insurance, and outcome evaluation. *Journal of the American Medical Association* 284: 1689–1695.

16. *Ibid.*

17. *Ibid.*

18. H. Fingarette, 1988. *Heavy drinking: The myth of alcoholism as a disease.* Berkeley, CA: University of California.

19. S. Peele, 1989. *Diseasing of America: Addiction treatment out of control.* Lexington, MA: Lexington Books.

20. S. Peele, 1988. On the diseasing of America. *Utne Reader* 30: p. 67.

21. H. Fingarette, 1988. *Heavy drinking: The myth of alcoholism as a disease.* Berkley, CA: University of California, p. 27.

22. G. E. Vailant, 1983. *The natural history of alcoholism.* Cambridge, MA: Harvard University Press, p. 309.

23. J. E. Royce, 1989. *Alcohol problems and alcoholism: A comprehensive survey* (Rev. ed.). New York: The Free Press, p. 89.

24. H. Fingarette, 1988. *Heavy drinking: The myth of alcoholism as a disease.* Berkeley, CA: University of California, p. 31.

25. Alcoholics Anonymous World Services, Inc., 1981. *Twelve steps and twelve traditions.* New York: Alcoholics Anonymous World Services, p. 5.

26. H. Fingarette, 1988. *Heavy drinking: The myth of alcoholism as a disease.* Berkeley, CA: University of California.

27. *Ibid.*

28. S. Peele, 1989. *Diseasing of America: Addiction treatment out of control.* Lexington, MA: Lexington Books.

29. G. A. Marlatt, B. Demming, & J. B. Reid, 1973. Loss of control drinking in alcoholics: An experimental analogue. *Journal of Abnormal Psychology* 81: 223–241.

30. J. E. Royce, 1989. *Alcohol problems and alcoholism: A comprehensive survey* (Rev. ed.). New York: The Free Press, p. 135.

31. M. Keller, 1972. On the loss-of-control phenomenon in alcoholism. *British Journal of Psychiatry* 67: 153–166.

32. H. Fingarette, 1988. *Heavy drinking: The myth of alcoholism as a disease.* Berkeley, CA: University of California, p. 44.

33. J. E. Royce, 1989. *Alcohol problems and alcoholism: A comprehensive survey* (Rev. ed.). New York: The Free Press, p. 123.

34. *Ibid.*

35. G. A. Marlatt & J. R. Gordon (Eds.), 1985. *Relapse prevention: Maintenance strategies in the treatment of addictive behaviors.* New York: Guildford Press, p. 7.

36. W. R. Miller & R. K. Hester, 1995. Treatment for alcohol problems: Toward an informed eclecticism. In R. K. Hester & W. R. Miller (Eds.). *Handbook of alcoholism treatment approaches: Effective alternatives* (2nd ed., pp. 1–11). Boston: Allyn & Bacon.

37. The information in this section is from Addiction: "Drugs, Brains, and Behavior—The Science of Addiction" published by the National Institute on Drug Abuse. http://www.drugabuse.gov/ScienceofAddiction/ (accessed January 7, 2010), p. 3.

38. Alcoholics Anonymous World Services Inc., 2008. *Alcoholics anonymous* (4th ed.). New York: Alcoholics Anonymous World Services, p. 30.

39. Alcoholics Anonymous World Services, Inc., 1981. *Twelve steps and twelve traditions.* New York: Alcoholics Anonymous World Services.

CHAPTER 3

1. American Psychiatric Association, 2000. *Diagnostic and statistical manual of mental disorders* (Fourth Edition, Text Revision). Washington, DC: American Psychiatric Association, p. 685.

2. *Ibid.*, p. 706.

3. *Ibid.*, p. 702.

4. J. Paris, 2004. Personality disorders over time: Implications for psychotherapy. *American Journal of Psychotherapy* 58: 420–429.

5. D. W. Black, 2000. Treatment for antisocial personality disorder. Psych Central. 2010. http://psychcentral.com/library/asp_tx.htm (accessed January 22, 2010), p. 2.

6. J. W. Dilley, 2004. Antisocial personality disorder. MedlinePlus Medical Encyclopedia. http://www.nlm.nih.gov/medlineplus/ency/article/000921.htm (accessed January 22, 2010).

7. Center for Substance Abuse Treatment, 2005. *Substance abuse treatment for persons with co-occurring disorders.* Treatment Improvement Protocol (TIP) Series 42. DHHS Publication No. (SMA) 05-3992. Rockville, MD: Substance Abuse and Mental Health Services Administration.

8. Office of Applied Studies, Substance Abuse and Mental Health Services Administration, 2009. Treatment Episode Data Set (TEDS). Highlights for 2007 Treatment Episode Data Set (TEDS). Table 2A: Admissions by primary substance of abuse, according to gender, race/ethnicity, and age at admission: TEDS 2007. http://wwwdasis.samhsa.gov/teds07/tedshigh2k7.pdf (accessed January 22, 2010).

9. Office of Applied Studies, Substance Abuse and Mental Health Services Administration, 2009. Treatment Episode Data Set (TEDS). Highlights for 2007 Treatment Episode Data Set (TEDS). Table 4: Admissions by primary substance of abuse, according to type of service, source of referral to treatment, and opioid replacement therapy: TEDS 2007. http://wwwdasis.samhsa.gov/teds07/tedshigh2k7.pdf (accessed January 22, 2010).

10. Office of Applied Studies, Substance Abuse and Mental Health Services Administration, 2009. Treatment Episode Data Set (TEDS) 2006: Discharges from Substance Abuse Treatment Services. Table 4: Admissions by primary substance of abuse, according to type of service, source of referral to treatment, and opioid replacement therapy: TEDS 2007. http://wwwdasis.samhsa.gov/teds06/teds2k6aweb508.pdf (accessed January 22, 2010).

11. Office of Applied Studies, Substance Abuse and Mental Health Services Administration, 2009. Treatment Episode Data Set (TEDS) 2006: Discharges from Substance Abuse Treatment Services. Table 3.2a: Admissions by primary substance of abuse, according to age of admission: TEDS 2006. http://wwwdasis.samhsa.gov/teds06/teds2k6aweb508.pdf (accessed January 22, 2010).

12. Office of Applied Studies, Substance Abuse and Mental Health Services Administration, 2009. Treatment Episode Data Set (TEDS) 2006: Discharges from Substance Abuse Treatment Services. http://wwwdasis.samhsa.gov/teds06/teds2k6aweb508.pdf (accessed January 22, 2010).

13. D. A. Regier, M. E. Farmer, D. S. Rae, B. Z. Locke, S. J. Keith, et al. 1990. Comorbidity of mental disorders with alcohol and other drug abuse: Results from the Epidemiologic Catchment (ECA) study. *JAMA* 264: 2511–2518.

14. Office of Applied Studies, Substance Abuse and Mental Health Services Administration, 2009. Treatment Episode Data Set (TEDS) 2006: Discharges from Substance Abuse Treatment Services. Table 2.4: Discharges in 2006 by type of service and reason for discharge: TEDS 2006. http://wwwdasis.samhsa.gov/teds06/tedsd2k6_508.pdf (accessed January 26, 2010).

15. Office of Applied Studies, Substance Abuse and Mental Health Services Administration, 2009. Treatment Episode Data Set (TEDS) 2006: Discharges from Substance Abuse Treatment Services. Table 2.7: Discharges in 2006, by characteristics at admission and type of service: TEDS 2006. http://wwwdasis.samhsa.gov/teds06/tedsd2k6_508.pdf (accessed January 26, 2010).

16. *Ibid.*

17. S. Fazel & J. Danesh, 2002. Serious mental disorder in 23,000 prisoners: A systematic review of 62 surveys. *The Lancet* 359: 545–550.

18. G. Cote & S. Hodgins, 1992. The prevalence of major mental disorders among homicide offenders. *International Journal of Law and Psychiatry* 15: 89–99.

CHAPTER 4

1. N. M. Petry, F. S. Stinson, & B. F. Grant, 2005. Comorbidity of DSM-IV pathological gambling and other psychiatric disorders: Results from the National Epidemiologic Survey on Alcohol and Related Conditions. *Journal of Clinical Psychiatry* 66: 564–574.

CHAPTER 5

1. Office of Applied Studies, Substance Abuse and Mental Health Services Administration, 2009. National Survey on Drug Use & Health. Table G.22—Cigarette Use in Lifetime, Past Year, and Past Month, by Detailed Age Category: Percentages, 2007 and 2008. http://oas.samhsa.gov/nsduh/2k8nsduh/AppG.htm#TabG-22 (accessed June 28, 2010)

2. National Academy of Sciences, 2003. *Reducing underage drinking: A collective responsibility.* Washington, DC: National Academic Press.

3. Center for Substance Abuse Treatment, 2005. *Substance abuse treatment for persons with co-occurring disorders.* Treatment Improvement Protocol (TIP) Series 42. DHHS Publication No. (SMA) 05-3992. Rockville, MD: Substance Abuse and Mental Health Services Administration.

4. W. White, 1998. *Slaying the dragon: The history of addiction treatment and recovery in America.* Bloomington, IL: Chestnut Health Systems/Lighthouse Institute.

5. Center for Substance Abuse Treatment, Substance Abuse and Mental Health Services Administration, no date. Screening, Brief Intervention, and Referral to Treatment. http://sbirt.samhsa.gov/index.htm (accessed November 19, 2010).

6. National Institute on Alcohol Abuse and Alcoholism, 2005. *Helping patients who drink too much: A clinician's guide.* NIH Publication No. 07-3769.

7. M. F. Fleming, M. P. Mundt, M. T. French, L. B. Manwell, E. A. Staauffacher, & K. L. Barry, 2002. Brief physician advice for problem drinkers: Long-term efficacy and cost-benefit analysis. *Alcoholism: Clinical and Experimental Research* 26: 36–43.

APPENDIX 1

1. Centers for Disease Control and Prevention, 2010. Alcohol & Public Health. http://www.cdc.gov/alcohol/ (accessed December 16, 2010).

2. Substance Abuse and Mental Health Services Administration, Office of Applied Studies, 2010. *Drug Abuse Warning Network, 2007: National Estimates of Drug-Related Emergency Department Visits.* https://dawninfo.samhsa.gov/files/ED2007/DAWN2k7ED.pdf (accessed December 16, 2010).

3. H. Harwood, 2000. Updating estimates of the economic costs of alcohol abuse in the United States: Estimates, update, methods, and data. National Institute on Alcohol Abuse and Alcoholism. http://pubs .niaaa.nih.gov/publications/economic-2000/alcoholcost.PDF (accessed December 16, 2010).

4. Substance Abuse and Mental Health Services Administration, Office of Applied Studies, 2010. *Drug Abuse Warning Network, 2007: National Estimates of Drug-Related Emergency Department Visits.* https://dawninfo.samhsa.gov/files/ED2007/DAWN2k7ED.pdf (accessed December 16, 2010).

5. Centers for Disease Prevention and Control, 2010. Chronic Disease Prevention and Health Promotion, Tobacco Use, Targeting the Nation's Leading Killer: At a Glance 2010. http://www.cdc.gov/chronicdisease/ resources/publications/aag/osh.htm (accessed December 16, 2010).

6. Substance Abuse and Mental Health Services Administration, Office of Applied Studies, 2010. *Drug Abuse Warning Network, 2007: National Estimates of Drug-Related Emergency Department Visits.* https://dawninfo.samhsa.gov/files/ED2007/DAWN2k7ED.pdf (accessed December 16, 2010).

7. Office of Applied Studies, Substance Abuse and Mental Health Services Administration, 2010. Results from the 2009 National Survey on Drug Use & Health: Detailed Tables. http://oas.samhsa.gov/NSDUH/ 2k9NSDUH/tabs/Sect1peTabs24to28.pdf (accessed December 16, 2010)

8. Substance Abuse and Mental Health Services Administration, Office of Applied Studies, 2010. *Drug Abuse Warning Network, 2007:*

National Estimates of Drug-Related Emergency Department Visits.
https://dawninfo.samhsa.gov/files/ED2007/DAWN2k7ED.pdf (accessed
December 16, 2010).

APPENDIX 2

1. S. T. Higgins, A. J. Budney, H. K. Bickel, G. Badger, F. Foerg, &
D. Ogden, 1995. Outpatient behavioral treatment for cocaine dependence:
One-year outcome. *Experimental & Clinical Psychopharmacology* 3:
205–212.

Index

About the Author

Gary L. Fisher is the founder, first director, and now a professor at the Center for the Application of Substance Abuse Technologies at the University of Nevada, Reno. Formerly a professor of Counseling and Educational Psychology, he is the author of a textbook on substance abuse counseling that is now in its fourth edition and *Rethinking Our War on Drugs: Candid Talk About Controversial Issues* published by Praeger. In addition, Fisher is the senior editor of an encyclopedia on substance abuse prevention, treatment, and recovery published in 2009. During his 36-year professional career, Fisher has worked as a private practice clinician and public school psychologist, as well as working 27 years as a university professor.